Dr.

DR MIKE SMITH
cine, a practisin ....ncaster and
writer. He was the Chief Medical Officer of the
Family Planning Association 1970–75 and their
Honorary Medical Adviser 1975–90. For many
years he has been a 'resident' expert guest on
BBC2's Jimmy Young Programme and was LBC's
regular broadcasting doctor from its inception and
continues with its successor, London News Talk
Radio. He has been seen and heard on most TV
channels and radio stations throughout the British
Isles over the last 25 years. In April 1991, he was
voted the TV and Radio Doctors' 'Expert's Expert'
in the *Observer* magazine's series.

His other books include *Birth Control, How to
Save Your Child's Life, A New Dictionary of Symptoms,
Dr Mike Smith's Handbook of Over-The-Counter
Medicines, Dr Mike Smith's First Aid Handbook* and
Dr Mike Smith's Handbook of Prescription Medicine.

IONA SMITH is a qualified nurse who has special-
ised in Family Planning and the menopause. She is
also a successful journalist. For many years she
wrote the medical page and answered readers'
letters for *Woman's Weekly* magazine, and previously co-wrote HRT. She therefore has special
knowledge and understanding of the problems
that concern women. She is married to Dr Mike
Smith and they have three grown-up children.

Also in *Dr Mike Smith's Postbag* series:

DR MIKE SMITH'S POSTBAG

INFERTILITY

DR MIKE SMITH
IONA SMITH

WITH SHARRON KERR

KYLE CATHIE LIMITED

Dr Mike Smith and Iona Smith are hereby identified as authors
of this work in accordance with Section 77 of the Copyright,
Designs and Patents Act 1988.

First published 1995 by
Kyle Cathie Limited
20 Vauxhall Bridge Road
London SW1V 2SA

ISBN 1 85626 202 2

A CIP catalogue record for this title
is available from the British Library

Typeset in Palatino by SX Composing Ltd, Rayleigh, Essex
Printed and bound in Great Britain by Cox & Wyman Ltd, Reading

CONTENTS

INTRODUCTION

The World Health Organisation has estimated that around one in ten of all couples in the world are infertile. However, the hard facts are that as many as one in six couples will experience fertility problems at some stage in their lives. While advances in medical science mean that now, more than ever before, there is hope that many fertility problems can be resolved, infertility and its treatment can bring heartbreak and suffering to even the strongest and most capable of couples. Treatment offers hope, but does not always bring success, and it can be a harrowing process for many couples. Dealing with waiting lists, appointment after appointment, constant trips to fertility centres, hopes being raised and then dashed, can never be easy.

The bitter disappointment of infertility often has a knock-on effect on personal relationships. Sexual relationships can become damaged. Family relationships may suffer too. Some couples become so depressed their marriage can irretrievably break down, adding to their loss of hope for the future and compounding their feelings of failure. They become understandably obsessed with trying to achieve a pregnancy, to the point where nothing else counts. Sadly, sometimes that very obsession, the striving to become pregnant, can be counter-productive. Stress alone can be sufficient to prevent, or at least seriously to delay, a pregnancy.

Of course, infertility can be due to a number of

factors other than stress. For example, scar tissue can build up, causing the 'kinking' of Fallopian tubes and thus preventing the egg from travelling down to be fertilised. It may be caused by hormonal problems, a low sperm count or inactive sperm in the man, or by dietary or health deficiencies. Some couples, who quickly have a first child without any difficulty and never imagine they may encounter subsequent problems, can nevertheless find it impossible to enlarge their family when they want to.

If treatment is unsuccessful, some couples are never able to come to terms with facing life without a child of their own. The ironic thing is that subfertility is one of the most common of all health problems, yet one that few really consider until it happens to them. Possibly because of this, those of us who find we can have children easily, almost without thought, often do not understand the significant psychological damage and pain, both mental and physical (in terms of treatment), that infertility can cause.

Thousands upon thousands of couples seek treatment in order to have the child they long for. Thankfully for many of those couples, who once had no chance whatsoever of having a child of their own, advances in medical science mean that they can now be given hope, and eventually in many cases produce the child they have so desperately wanted.

There can be no denying that the new advances in infertility treatment are exceptional. Further good news is that British scientists and doctors have been involved in the front line of this pioneering work. Research is breaking new ground all the time as newer and newer discoveries are made.

These days IVF (*in vitro* fertilisation, or 'test-tube' babies) is an accepted term with few people ignorant of its meaning, yet only twenty years ago this treatment was unheard of. The use of hormones to stimulate the ovaries and ultrasound to monitor the response from the ovary, the process of IVF itself, the carrying out of microsurgery for tubal disease, the development of sperm injection techniques and the screening of embryos to improve IVF and reduce miscarriage, have all brought enormous benefits in treating infertility.

With all the high-tech advances it is little wonder that many couples are confused about the options available to them. It would be impossible in a book of this nature and size to cover every aspect of infertility in detail. What I aim to do, therefore, is to give the reader an overview of infertility and to set out clearly and simply what infertility means, how you can boost your chances of conception if you are trying for a baby, and to explain briefly what treatment is on offer for those whose conception difficulties are persisting. I also give examples of questions I am often asked.

My aim in writing this book is that being more informed makes you forearmed and consequently more able to deal with the difficult journey to parenthood or trying to come to terms with a life without children. Knowledge can also help you to fight your corner more effectively; by knowing what treatment is available, you will be able to choose the best for you. Also, being forearmed with information, you will perhaps have the confidence to ask more questions of the medical staff with whom you come into contact.

PREPARING FOR CONCEPTION

Conception is not as simple as it seems. While fertility problems may affect one in six couples, even those couples who do not appear to have any difficulties will only have a likelihood of between one in four and one in five of conceiving each month. The other interesting thing about this statistic is that it is not greatly different from the success rates of most assisted conception methods. And even when a woman has conceived and missed her first period, it is not one hundred per cent certain that the pregnancy will be successful – at this stage the chances are seventy-two per cent.

The route from sperm to egg can be a tricky one with problems arising at every stage. A woman is born with some 500,000 eggs in her ovaries. At the beginning of each cycle about twenty-nine eggs begin to grow in the ovary, yet only one reaches maturity and is subsequently released for possible fertilisation.

A man on the other hand produces new sperm all the time. The quality of the sperm can be affected, for good or ill, by current circumstances and it is therefore important to look at your lifestyle and general health when thinking about planning a baby. Illness, exposure to radiation, smoking or heavy drinking, for example, may have a harmful effect, or a healthy lifestyle may bring benefits. New sperm take about seventy-two days to develop to maturity in the testes; even fertile men will have some unhealthy or deformed

sperm. In some instances an egg may be successfully fertilised by the man's sperm, but
subsequently will fail to implant in the womb.
Some figures suggest that as many as eight out of
ten fertilised eggs can be lost in this way.

If you are trying for a baby it may be helpful to
understand how you can improve your fertility
and when you are at your most fertile.

WHAT IS INFERTILITY?

Many people fail to realise that the averagely fertile
couple having intercourse during the most fertile
part of the monthly cycle has, at best, only a one in
four chance of producing a baby.

It may be reassuring for some readers to understand that infertility is not a black and white,
clear-cut issue. The International Health Foundation points out that more than two-thirds of those
diagnosed as 'infertile' are actually sub-fertile, and
can be helped by assisted conception treatments.
Very few couples – fewer than five per cent – are
actually infertile. Most have conditions which
make them sub-fertile and within this category
there are various degrees of sub-fertility, including
some where there are chances, albeit very small
ones, of conceiving naturally. This view is empha-
sised by John Dickson, executive director of ISSUE,
the National Fertility Association.

> If you took 100 people on day one, at the end
> of the year 90 would have conceived. 10
> would not and out of those 10 only half
> would conceive over the next year. Infertility
> is a sliding scale from the very fecund –
> people who fall pregnant straight away – to

the completely sterile. There is a sort of grey patch in the middle of people who could conceive and may conceive if left to their own devices – although it may take them something like seven years to do so.

From the medical point of view, whether or not a couple's failure to conceive may need investigation and/or treatment, infertility tends to be defined as the inability to conceive after having regular and unprotected sex two or three times a week for more than a year without a pregnancy occurring.

When should you start to worry?

How long does it take to conceive? Many couples, often after years of taking contraceptive precautions, expect to get pregnant immediately once those precautions are abandoned. Contrary to popular opinion and news reports about the world's ever increasing population, man is one of the least fertile of all animals. While it is only natural that you may start to feel anxious if pregnancy doesn't occur within a month or so, it is important to remember, as I've already explained, that it can take several months or even longer than that to become pregnant when there are absolutely no fertility problems. Even couples who already have children may find difficulty in conceiving again, so although failure to become pregnant quickly is indeed distressing, it is not uncommon.

The normal guidance when a couple fail to conceive is that they should seek medical advice after a year of trying if they are under thirty, and after six months if they are over thirty.

When a couple cannot conceive and tests show there is something physically wrong with one partner, it is usually about fifty-fifty as to whether the problem is with the man or woman. Other interpretations suggest that a third of fertility problems can be attributed to a woman, a further third to the man and the remaining third to a combination of both partners, for example, endometriosis in the woman (see page 26) and a low sperm count in the man.

If you have been trying to get pregnant for a few months without success, generally at this stage there should not be cause for too much concern. Nevertheless, there are instances when you should consult your GP sooner rather than later. These include if either partner believes that there could be any reason for infertility problems, such as a history of sexually transmitted disease, or conditions known to be associated with infertility in the woman. These include endometriosis or pelvic inflammatory disease, pelvic or abdominal surgery which may have led to scarring or adhesions, kinking or sticking to the pelvic organs, or a history of hormonal problems. The latter may prevent ovulation and thus stop the period or cause very irregular cycles. Other medical causes which might affect fertility are diabetes, an under-functioning thyroid or kidneys, gross overdieting causing extreme thinness or the other extreme, gross obesity.

Age, too, is another factor that you should consider. John Dickson, of ISSUE, strongly believes that the age of a woman is critical in terms of her fertility.

Men can be potent at sixty, but with women it's a biological fact that between thirty-five and forty fertility rates start to turn down,

and post forty they drop off quite dramatically. So if you leave having children until
your mid thirties, you are taking a gamble.

A healthy woman of forty may take twice as long
to conceive as her twenty-year-old counterpart. It
is well known that the ability to conceive dimin-
ishes markedly over the age of forty-five and a
large proportion of women who are still men-
struating at fifty will find it extremely difficult to
conceive. Pregnancies when a woman is in her
forties are now commonplace, but should a pregnancy occur at fifty plus, it brings with it a set of
problems for the older mother. Chances of a rise in
blood pressure, for example, or prolongation of the
time spent in labour are increased in the later fertile years. There is also an increased risk of
diabetes, thrombosis, toxaemia of pregnancy or
heart disease associated with pregnancy. More
specifically, the chances of the baby having a
genetic abnormality do rise quite markedly when
a woman is over forty.

You can take heart from the fact that, according
to the International Health Foundation, which per-
forms research and provides information in the
fields of family planning, menopause and in-
voluntary childlessness, as many as one in four
women seeking medical advice for infertility
become pregnant during investigations.

HOW TO IMPROVE YOUR CHANCES OF CONCEPTION

Taking a healthy approach to the preparation for
pregnancy is known as preconceptual care. How
important is health before conception, you may

ask? The answer is that it does play a part in fertility. You do improve the likelihood of conception and a healthy baby by improving your own health before deciding you want to become pregnant or to father a child.

There are several factors that can affect fertility for both men and women. Among these are:

- *Smoking.* Cigarettes are thought to be one of the worst pollutants we come across. They contain hydrocarbons, carbon-monoxide, nicotine and nitrogen-dioxide. Apart from the damage smoking does to your own general health, smoking is also associated with fertility problems in men as it may damage sperm. Men who smoke tend to produce fewer sperm and have more damaged sperm. Female smokers run twice the risk of miscarriage or premature delivery.
- *Drinking too much alcohol.* Occasional social and really temperate drinking is likely to be harmless, but many, if not most, mothers-to-be will often be cautious and stop drinking altogether. Heavy drinking can also affect a woman's menstrual cycle. Alcohol is a substance that is frequently ignored when men are thinking about fatherhood. However, it is a powerful sperm toxicant. Many men find that their sperm counts improve dramatically when they give up drinking alcohol for a minimum of three months. Sperm are very sensitive and there is much evidence that alcohol dampens fertility.
- *Certain prescribed drugs* (anti-depressants, for example) can decrease sperm production, so if you have to take medicines and are thinking about trying to start a family, do discuss this with your GP. It is important to check whether the medication

you are prescribed could affect your fertility or the health of a future pregnancy.

Over the Counter medicines (commonly known as OTCs) are widely taken by men and women. Keeping to the recommended dose and only taking such medicines when they are essential is good advice for everyone to follow, especially prospective parents, lest the chance of conception or implantation is reduced.

More worrying are the 'social' drugs, such as cannabis, cocaine and the amphetamine-like compounds. No one is sure of the extent of their use, but my postbag regularly contains letters from worried women who were taking these drugs before they discovered their pregnancy. Except with excessive use or the abuse of hard drugs, the individual risk is not greatly increased. However, no one knows how damaging such 'social' use is in reducing the chances of conception.

● *Workplace hazards.* Exposure to radiation and some workplace chemicals could also be possible causes of infertility. If you do work with dangerous materials, always follow any safety guidelines advised.

PREPARING FOR PREGNANCY

So what other areas of your life do you need to concentrate on to increase your fertility by improving your general health?

Medical check-up

You can start by visiting your doctor for a health check to see that your blood pressure is normal and that you are not unhealthily overweight. Your doctor may order blood tests, for example, to check that you are not anaemic or to find out whether or not you are protected against rubella (German measles). This is particularly important if you are starting infertility treatment to become pregnant. If treatment were successful it would be very unfortunate to contract rubella during the first three months of pregnancy and then be faced with the dilemma of having to decide on termination because of possible foetal damage. If you are not immune, you will be offered a vaccination and be advised not to get pregnant for the next three months.

Diet
You can look at your diet and think about whether you are eating healthily. Stop smoking, cut down on alcohol and also cut down on drinks containing caffeine. Tests have shown that too much coffee or other caffeine drinks can reduce a woman's fertility as well as affect a baby's birth weight.

Maintaining normal body weight is important. Being underweight, or having anorexia nervosa, can mean that your periods stop and being obese can affect fertility too. In conditions such as the polycystic ovary syndrome – when a woman's ovaries have many cysts that can make her less fertile than usual – being heavily overweight may be the 'final straw'. The excess fat tissue itself produces hormones which prevent the woman's ovaries from functioning as well as they would otherwise. Miscarriage is also more likely in those women who are seriously overweight.

Maintaining a healthy diet applies to men as well as women. Eating plenty of fruit and vegetables enhances the levels of minerals and Vitamins A, C and E in the body, which are thought to play a part in improving sperm quality.

Stress avoidance

Taking exercise can help you get fit and is a good way of dealing with stress. Too much anxiety may prevent a woman from ovulating. It is also thought that stress can affect sperm production. Men should not underestimate their emotional state of mind if there is a delay in conceiving. Talking honestly about how they are feeling may help them deal with stress as well.

Folic acid supplements

Women thinking about getting pregnant should take a folic acid supplement. Folic acid, part of the Vitamin B complex, is essential for growth and blood formation. There is evidence to suggest that it might help prevent spina bifida – a neural tube defect – if taken by women before conception. At the end of 1992 the Chief Medical Officer asked doctors to advise all women who were planning a pregnancy in the near future to take 0.4 mg of folic acid daily before trying to conceive and until the twelfth week of pregnancy.

Coming off the Pill

Women often ask me when they should stop taking the Pill. Should you stop taking the Pill for three months before you try to conceive and why? The Pill does not have a lasting effect on fertility, although after some women stop taking it, they may experience a short delay of a month or two before they are able to get pregnant. The general consensus seems to be that if you have used contraceptives in the past the chances of sub-sequently having a successful pregnancy are not reduced because of that factor alone. Some doctors consider it ideal to switch to another method of contraception such as the cap or condom for three months before trying to get pregnant. This should give your body's hormones and your menstrual cycle time to get back to normal, although there is no evidence that if you don't do this it is harmful.

Increasing the sperm count

It may be the subject of jokes but wearing tight underpants is not conducive to healthy sperm pro-duction. Nature did not intend testicles to become overheated which is why they are situated in a little sack outside the body – the scrotum. For the production of sperm a constant temperature is needed. This is why the scrotum hangs down away from the body when it is hot, and seems to shrink as it retracts towards the body for warmth when it is cold.

Tight underpants, tight trousers or tight Lycra cycling shorts can allow the testicles to become overheated, which in turn may affect sperm pro-duction and lower the number produced. Men should wear loose boxer shorts and avoid very hot baths. As sperm are produced constantly, a count that might have been lowered by excess heat can recover once the testicles are kept a degree or so below the temperature of the rest of the body. However, it will take a few weeks for the count to rise significantly. Being overweight can also make the temperature of the testicles too high for good sperm production.

There are doctors who believe that wearing loose pants or deliberately cooling the testicles has no

value. However, should a varicocoele be present –
a kind of varicose vein surrounding the scrotum –
its removal will increase sperm quantity and
quality. With any such scrotal abnormalities, such
as a protruding hernia, a doctor's examination and
advice is wise if not essential.

CONCEPTION

It is relevant here to discuss briefly a man and a woman's sexual organs so that you understand the way your own bodies work and you are familiar with terms that may be used when talking about fertility.

THE FEMALE REPRODUCTIVE SYSTEM

A woman's reproductive organs lie within the lower part of her body, protected by the bones of her pelvis.

There are two ovaries located either side of the womb. They are glands about the size of almonds, or the size of a thumbnail, which produce the eggs, or *ova*, and also the female sex hormones, oestrogen and progesterone. A woman is born with about 500,000 immature eggs (*ova*) in her ovaries. These lie dormant until puberty, which usually commences between the ages of ten and sixteen. Only a few hundred eggs will ever mature fully between puberty and the menopause, which generally occurs at between forty and fifty years of age.

The Fallopian tubes lead from the ovaries to the womb. At the ends of the tubes are finger-like structures which help to collect the eggs released by the ovaries.

The womb, or uterus, is about the size and shape of an upside-down pear, or a small adult fist. It is a very elastic muscular organ with thick, muscular walls able to stretch around a growing foetus. The lining of the womb (endometrium) is soft and filled with blood. Each month, when you are not pregnant, the lining is shed in your monthly period and then renewed.

The cervix is the base of the womb and it has a small, central opening known as the os. Blood comes through it during the monthly period, and sperm can swim up through it during intercourse. During labour, the cervix gradually opens up to allow the baby to be born.

The vagina is a stretchy tube some three inches long. From its opening in the vulva, it leads up to the cervix. The vaginal walls are soft and elastic, to enable them to stretch easily around a man's penis during intercourse or to accommodate a baby during labour.

THE MALE REPRODUCTIVE SYSTEM

The testicles produce the sperm which are needed to fertilise the woman's egg. They also produce the male sex hormones, of which testosterone is the most important. There are two testicles in the scrotum (a bag of skin) which are made up internally of one kilometre of fine tubes. The scrotum is situated outside the body, below the penis. One testicle usually hangs lower than the other. The testicles produce millions of sperm each day from puberty onwards. Sperm have a head, neck and tail, and can move by flicking the tail from side to side.

Sperm travel from the testicles by means of a tube, called the *vas deferens*, to the vesicles, where the seminal fluid, or semen, is produced. Sexual stimulation causes the tissue inside the penis to fill with blood, making the penis hard and erect. During sexual intercourse sperm are propelled along the urethra and ejaculated from the tip of the penis into the woman's vagina. In one ejaculation there are about 200 to 400 million sperm. Some sperm pass through the cervix into the womb. Passage through the cervical mucus helps to eliminate less vigorous or abnormal sperm. Sperm which progress into the womb retain their fertilising power for about two to three days.

THE MONTHLY CYCLE

A woman's monthly cycle usually lasts for twenty-eight days, although some have cycles a few days shorter and others a few days longer. The regular bleeding which occurs as part of this cycle is a very obvious sign that the cycle is drawing to a close. But ovulation is usually also a regular part of the cycle, although it is not so obvious. Ovulation is the medical name for the start of a woman's most fertile period. A woman ovulates – and is most likely to conceive – fourteen days before her period. It is quite a common falsehood that you ovulate fourteen days from the beginning of your period. This idea has probably arisen because we tend to talk of menstrual cycles in terms of twenty-eight days. But as cycles can vary from woman to woman the best way of working out when you ovulate is to count back from the first day of your period. Women who may be having problems conceiving ask me whether the length of their menstrual cycle has anything to do with it. This worry is unfounded because the length of the cycle alone, if it is within the usual 'normal' range of twenty-one to thirty-two days, does not affect the ability to conceive.

But how can you tell when this is happening? Some women know when they are about to ovulate just by 'listening' to their bodies. They actually feel a slight cramping pain, similar to a period pain, when the egg is released.

Others notice physical changes in the cervical mucus which protects the womb from infection. The everyday discharge that most women experience is due to the natural secretions in the cervical canal, as well as the secretory cells that produce a lubricating moisture when a woman is sexually aroused. Although these natural secretions are usually white, they can vary in amount and texture at different times of the month.

Not all women find these mucus changes easy to spot. Some will only notice a small amount of milky wetness for a few days, which disappears after ovulation. As ovulation approaches, more mucus is produced and it becomes thinner and clearer, which makes it easier for the sperm to pass through. So when you are ovulating the mucus will be clear, and can be stretched between your thumb and forefinger almost like a piece of elastic. After ovulation the mucus becomes thick and opaque.

If you do start looking at your bodily changes in this way you will probably recognise your own signs fairly quickly. You could even make a note of any change in cervical mucus on the same chart that you log your temperature (see details of temperature charting on page 19).

Calculating the fertile period within the monthly cycle

You can keep a note of your periods and work out how long your cycle seems to be. If your cycle is extremely regular, you will be able to work out roughly when you are ovulating by counting back fourteen days from the beginning of your period. However, if you do want to know precisely when you are ovulating, buy an extra-sensitive thermometer or hormone-testing kit, which is more accurate, from your pharmacist.

If you wish you can detect the time of the month when you are most fertile by using a sensitive thermometer. When you are ovulating, your temperature rises slightly. The thermometer will show a slight change, a little rise in the temperature of no more than 0.2°C or 0.4°F, which means that you have just ovulated. You will need to take your temperature every morning. If you keep this up regularly and chart the results, you may see a pattern emerging. This will help you to predict when you are going to ovulate and thus when would be the best time – in terms of trying to conceive – for sex.

Women ask me why they need to take their temperatures first thing in the morning rather than another time of day. The basal body temperature (BBT) is the temperature of the body at complete rest. Over the course of the monthly cycle, hormonal changes produce slight fluctuations in that temperature. Taking the temperature later in the day will reflect other factors, which are not relevant to the fertility cycle.

Hormone-testing kits are used upon the urine. They tend to show that ovulation is probably going to happen during the next twenty-four to thirty-six hours, rather than pinpointing the exact moment of ovulation.

The hormones needed for the maturation and development of an egg-containing follicle in the ovary, and the releasing of a matured egg, are called the follicle stimulating hormone (FSH) and the luteinising hormone (LH). Hormone-testing kits work by measuring the amount of the hormone that triggers ovulation. Just before ovulation your urine contains a higher level of this hormone.

HOW CONCEPTION TAKES PLACE

A woman is most likely to conceive if she has intercourse around the time she ovulates – that is, when an egg is released from one of her ovaries. An egg lives for only about a day, though sperm survive in good numbers for about two to three days, so there is only a short time in each month when conception is possible. If you are having regular sex two or three times each week you are sure to include the period around ovulation, which is the best time to conceive.

The sperm swim into the womb and on into the Fallopian tubes. When an egg is released by the ovary, the fingers at the end of the Fallopian tube help to direct the egg down into the tube. Simultaneously, hormones produced by the ovaries cause the lining of the womb to begin to thicken and fill with blood. It is in one of the Fallopian tubes that the egg is usually fertilised. Chemicals released by the egg attract the sperm and a number will cluster around it. But only one out of all the millions of sperm originally ejaculated joins with the egg to fertilise it. The time taken from ejaculation to fertilisation is usually no more than about an hour.

Over a period of days after fertilisation, the egg continues to travel down the Fallopian tube. Eventually it reaches the uterus or womb, where it attaches itself to the soft lining, which has thickened in order to receive a fertilised egg. The fertilised egg will embed itself within this enriched lining for nourishment during the early days of pregnancy. This is called implantation, and once this has happened conception is said to have taken place. If the egg is not fertilised it will die and, together with the now unwanted lining, will be discharged via the vagina as the blood and tissue fluids which make up a period. After this, the cycle begins again.

How often should you have intercourse?

Some people argue that you should have intercourse less often because they believe that the more a man ejaculates, the smaller is the number of sperm produced.

Research has shown that the previous advice of 'saving it up' and then having intercourse around the time of ovulation has no real benefits. It may in fact have disadvantages, because it can make a couple over-anxious. It is now considered that 'saving it up' does not improve semen quality and may even cause a decline if ejaculation doesn't take place every couple of days.

Women can predict the most fertile period in their monthly cycle by keeping a temperature chart or using a hormone-testing kit (see page 19), and increase the chances of conception by having intercourse at this time. Working out when you are ovulating should not be used for a long time without getting proper medical advice. And certainly if you do try to work out when you are ovulating, and suspect that you might not, after all, be ovulating, do seek your GP's advice.

However, being too concerned about the precise moment of ovulation can turn lovemaking into a chore and cause unnecessary anxiety, which itself can prevent conception. Couples trying for a baby are now usually advised to have intercourse just as regularly as they want to, between every one to three days, and not to try to target precisely the day a woman is most likely to ovulate – fourteen days before her next period. If you make love fairly frequently it is less difficult to miss ovulation. And it is also worth remembering that sperm do remain active in a woman's body for up to three days.

IF NOTHING HAPPENS, WHAT'S THE NEXT STEP?

Quite understandably, having a failure to conceive investigated can be difficult to deal with and some people may be reluctant to seek medical help. However, remember that some problems can be treated fairly straightforwardly and could save you months of worry and anxiety. If you are worried do seek the help of your GP. He or she will be able to explain to you anything you don't fully understand and can arrange, if necessary, for the first investigations – such as sperm and blood tests – to be undertaken.

You will need a letter of referral from your GP in order to be referred to a fertility specialist. There are many possible reasons for an infertility problem, and as the difficulty may lie with one or other, or perhaps both partners, the couple will usually be seen together at their first visit to the fertility clinic. See also the chapter on dealing with your doctor (page 70).

THE CAUSES OF INFERTILITY

Infertility is a common problem caused by a wide variety of factors, some of which may be difficult to pinpoint initially, and some of which may never be discovered. Often there can be one or more problems existing together or a problem in both male and female partners. As a very general rule, a couple should consider they have a problem if they fail to conceive for up to a year. Mischance alone may be the reason, but in couples who are over thirty, or when external anxieties about the delay are adding to the problem, some investigations may be started earlier.

Infections

Fertility problems in both sexes can sometimes be due to infections such as sexually transmitted disease – the one due to the *Chlamydia* germ in particular, especially in the female partner. So if you think you could have an infection do get your symptoms checked and dealt with by your GP before any serious damage occurs.

INFERTILITY IN WOMEN

Fallopian tube problems

In women a blockage in the Fallopian tubes is a common cause of infertility, possibly accounting for twenty to thirty per cent of all cases. Scar tissue can build up causing the 'kinking' of Fallopian tubes, preventing the egg from travelling down to be fertilised. Tubes may not be totally obstructed – in some cases they can just be scarred or stuck to nearby tissues so that eggs cannot get down them into the uterus.

Infection can damage the tube and a wide variety of different bacteria can cause damage. I am often asked whether blocked Fallopian tubes are always the result of a sexually transmitted disease or pelvic inflammatory disorder. The answer is mostly, but not always. Problems with the Fallopian tubes can be associated with inflammation in the abdomen or germs of a non-sexually transmitted nature. Either may have occurred years before the woman thinks about having children.

Ectopic pregnancy

An ectopic pregnancy may cause complications in terms of fertility. Once combined, the egg normally moves down, embeds in the wall of the uterus and continues to grow into a baby. With an ectopic pregnancy, however, the combined cells do not move on. The term 'ectopic pregnancy' itself literally means a pregnancy occurring in a place other than the womb. In practice, ectopic pregnancies mostly occur in one of the Fallopian tubes. The combined cells start to grow in the walls of the Fallopian tube. If not operated upon quickly, the egg will burst through the tube into the abdomen, usually resulting in the need to remove the affected tube. This still leaves the tube on the other side intact and, if it is healthy, a woman will still be able to get pregnant in the normal way.

Failure to ovulate due to hormone imbalance

Hormones such as adrenaline, insulin, oestrogen and testosterone, influence nearly every aspect of our lives: our growth, our emotions, menstrual cycle, sexual feelings and metabolism, for instance. Most hormones are produced by endocrine glands in the body, such as the pituitary, the thyroid, the adrenals, the pancreas, the ovaries and the testes, and are released directly into the blood stream. They interact with each other as the body's chemical messengers and normally a fine balance is achieved and controlled by a complex network of nerves. Such a complex system gives plenty of scope for things to go wrong.

The menstrual cycle is controlled by a complicated interplay of hormones. The first day of period bleeding is taken as the first day of the menstrual cycle. As the period progresses, the pituitary gland in the brain secretes a hormone called follicle stimulating hormone (FSH), which together with the hormone oestrogen (secreted by the ovaries), works to mature and ripen another immature egg ready for later ovulation.

A third hormone, called luteinising hormone (LH), is then responsible for ovulation, as it stimulates the release of the egg from the ovary. About a day before ovulation, there is a steep rise in the amount of LH in the body, known as the LH surge. After the egg has been released, the ovaries are triggered to produce another hormone, progesterone, which accelerates the development of the womb lining ready for implantation. If fertilisation has occurred and the egg has implanted, levels of progesterone will increase throughout pregnancy.

It is thought that in approximately four out of ten cases of female infertility there is a problem with ovulation or abnormal ovulatory function. Sometimes stopping taking the Pill, which regulates the reproductive hormones chemically, can temporarily interfere with ovulation and it may take a little while for the hormone system to settle down again. An injectable method of contraception can also interrupt ovulation patterns, as can stress and strenuous exercise.

There can be many other causes for such a problem, including low hormone excretion from the pituitary gland in the brain, polycystic ovaries (see page 11) and ovarian failure. Period problems and early menopause can be caused by hormonal disorders.

Weight problems
Strict dieting and being underweight, as well as being overweight, can also aggravate any problems with ovulation. Obesity can affect fertility. One specific connection is a condition called PCOS, Polycystic Ovary Syndrome (see page 11).

Endometriosis
The endometrium is the tissue that lines the uterus. Endometriosis is a strange but not uncommon condition whereby deposits of endometrial tissue occur outside the womb. The natural monthly hormones cause a build-up in the lining of the womb, in preparation for the fertilised egg. But when there is no fertilised egg, the hormone level plummets and the period starts. Unfortunately, the same hormone which causes the womb lining to build up and then fall away has a similar effect on endometrial tissue elsewhere. So, wherever the tissue has been misplaced, whether on the outside of the womb, on the ovary or Fallopian tube, a tiny bleed (like a period) occurs within that tissue.

The surrounding tissue to which the endometriosis is attached, as well as that of the endometriosis itself, can become inflamed. This causes swelling, pain and, within months, scar tissue can be formed. Fortunately, hormones can be prescribed to prevent periods for a time. With no period, there is no build-up of womb lining and, for the sufferer, no bleeding of the diseased tissue. When the hormone treatment is stopped after nine months, all may have quietened down so much that the symptoms disappear. But, if symptoms persist, the gynaecologist may suggest surgery to remove some endometriosis deposits. Nowadays this is usually done by laparoscopy. This means using a tube – called a laparoscope – and then often hot-wire diathermy or a laser beam as the 'instrument' of removal. Both seal the tissues as they remove the endometrial deposits, so making the process quick and efficient.

Most cases of endometriosis are mild, with no apparent symptoms. Often the problem is only detected during surgery for some other condition, or while investigating infertility which may have caused distress for many years.

Endometriosis can cause infertility although it is thought that some six out of ten women will be able to have children even after having hormone treatment. The remaining four out of ten cases may find they cannot conceive naturally. This is because adhesions caused by scar tissue may hinder the egg's progress between the ovary and the Fallopian tube.

Womb abnormalities and fibroids
A small proportion of female infertility is caused by congenital abnormalities (if you were born with a malformed uterus) or diseases of the womb.

Benign tumours called fibroids can cause infertility, as can abnormalities formed before birth, or damage and adhesions to the womb lining.

The walls of the womb are composed of elastic muscle tissue – enabling it to expand and contract during pregnancy and childbirth – interwoven with strengthening fibrous tissue. Sometimes, for unknown reasons, benign (non-cancerous) growths or 'knots' called fibroids form in this muscle tissue. Depending on their size and situation – submucous, subserous or intramural – they may or may not cause problems.

Fibroids seldom occur in women under thirty. They can be tiny and numerous (200 or more is not unknown) or can grow – usually very slowly – to reach the size of a large grapefruit. They rarely cause pain. Heavy, prolonged, or more frequent periods are their most common symptoms and 'flooding' can also be alarming. This excessive blood loss can, after several months, result in anaemia, tiredness and palpitations. Infertility can be associated with fibroids because a fibroid may be preventing implantation. Surgery to remove fibroids may be helpful.

Ovarian cysts

An ovarian cyst is a swelling in the ovary which can vary in size from just a few centimetres in diameter to be large enough to simulate pregnancy. If there are many of them in an ovary they may interfere with its production of hormones or ova, and so cause infertility.

Cervical problems

Cervical mucus can sometimes be too thick and the sperm cannot get through the cervix and into the womb. In rare cases the mucus – known in this

case as hostile cervical mucus – may contain antibodies which inactivate the sperm. Treatment is
usually artificial insemination directly into the
womb (IUI) or, in more serious cases, IVF.

Miscarriage

Women who can conceive but who miscarry re-
currently are considered technically to be infertile.
Miscarriage, also known by doctors as abortion
(whether it occurs unexpectedly or deliberately) is
very common indeed. Possibly as many as three
out of four conceptions end in this way. Studies
show that many miscarriages occur so early on that
the woman has not even missed a period or
realised she is pregnant. But at least one in six con-
firmed pregnancies ends in miscarriage, too. More
than half the women who miscarry will then go on
to have a normal healthy baby without any treatment at all.

Many miscarriages happen because something
goes wrong at a very early stage in the development of the foetus or the placenta.
Abnormalities occurring in the baby's genetic
make-up or in its developing heart or nervous
system are other likely causes. Some drugs or an
infection, such as rubella (German measles) or
heavy drinking or smoking, may cause abnormalities in the foetus and lead to miscarriage. Fibroids
or polyps (benign growths) which protrude into
the womb, or an intra-uterine contraceptive device
left in place during pregnancy, are amongst other
possible causes. Often however, particularly if
miscarriage occurs in the first three months of
pregnancy, the cause cannot be pinpointed.

In the second three months, miscarriage is much
less common and the cause is often apparent and

treatable – for example, an 'incompetent cervix' – which also accounts for many recurrent miscarriages. Normally, during pregnancy the cervical hole, which is the entrance to the womb, remains tightly closed until contractions in the first stage of labour dilate it to allow the baby through. With an incompetent cervix the hole is already slightly open, and the pressure on it as the baby grows larger increases the gap until the baby almost falls out. Once the problem has been diagnosed, the gynaecologist can insert a special stitch around the cervix for support – usually done about the fourteenth week of pregnancy – which is removed as the delivery date approaches.

Some repeated miscarriages are due to hormonal problems, most of which can be effectively treated with hormones, or by an abnormally shaped womb which is often treatable by surgery. In some women recurrent miscarriage may be due to their body's rejection of the foetus, similar to the rejection that can follow a kidney transplant. This was a particular problem until about forty years ago, when a mother with Rhesus negative blood could produce Rhesus antibodies if her developing baby's blood was Rhesus positive. This can now be prevented by giving a mother-to-be with Rhesus negative blood an injection of gammaglobulin at the time of the birth or miscarriage. This counteracts the Rhesus positive antigen – the common link that causes the Rhesus negative mother to produce antibodies that create subsequent obstetric problems.

When some women produce abnormal embryos leading to miscarriage, IVF may be a possible solution, since the embryo to be implanted is checked for abnormalities before implantation, making rejection far less likely.

Age

There is no doubt that age plays a role in a woman's fertility rate. Many women are deciding to start a family later on in life these days, usually because of career pressures, but you should bear in mind that if you choose to start a family in your mid thirties you are taking a gamble. Women are at their most fertile period, and therefore are most likely to conceive, somewhere around the age of twenty-four. Fertility declines from then on.

INFERTILITY IN MEN

Figures for male infertility range from three to five out of ten couples having problems conceiving. These are usually due to sperm abnormality, usually low sperm count or poor shape and swim-mability (motility). Less common causes include hormonal irregularities, or a gland such as the thyroid not working properly and so affecting the functioning of the testicles. The man may have antibodies against his own sperm, sometimes due to a previous infection or injury to the testicles (testes). In very rare cases there may be a problem of retrograde ejaculation, which means that the man ejaculates backwards into the bladder.

Low sperm count

A normally healthy man can produce at least 120 million sperm each time he ejaculates, although a count of just 100 million is also considered normal. This quantity is needed for the male to have the best chance of fertilising a single egg as a great many sperm die on the journey towards fer-tilisation. When a man has a low sperm count (oligospermia) of, say, 20 million sperm, he may not be very fertile.

The testicles are placed within the scrotum – outside the body – to keep them cool, and too many hot baths or the wearing of tight underpants may cause a reduction in the number of sperm produced in some men (see page 13). Likewise, a type of varicose vein around the testicles – a varicocoele – may be warming them more than nature intended. Surgical removal of the varicocele may correct the problem.

A bag of fluid found in the scrotum and surrounding the testes, known as a hydrocele, can also lower sperm production and may need to be surgically removed. A low sperm count can arise because of social factors, such as heavy drinking or taking anti-depressants. Often, however, there is no satisfactory explanation and, regrettably, no satisfactory way of increasing production.

Environmental factors are currently causing concern. Recent research has revealed that the average sperm count has halved in the last fifty years. The blame is pointed at environmental pollutants, ranging from pesticides, food additives or other chemicals called endocrine-disrupting chemicals. It is thought these could affect embryo development, for example the development of the testes in the womb. However, some researchers argue that there is little evidence that male fertility is declining and claim that male and female infertility rates appear constant over the last thirty years.

A low sperm count doesn't always mean that a man cannot make his wife pregnant without fertility treatment. In such cases it may just take the couple much longer to conceive.

Poor motility
Together with the problem of fewer sperm than average, there is the problem of poor sperm motility – or the way the sperm move. A word that you

may hear mentioned is asthenozoospermia, which simply means that more than four out of ten sperm have poor motility. This is a slightly more complicated problem than not producing enough sperm and IVF treatment may be advised.

Abnormal sperm

If more than a third of sperm look abnormal, infertility often results. Having too many abnormal sperm in the semen is sometimes referred to as teratozoospermia. When sperm are referred to as abnormal this means that they have poor shape and they are therefore unable to penetrate the egg's outer layer in order to fertilise it.

A high level of abnormal sperm doesn't mean that a subsequent pregnancy will be abnormal.

Antibodies

A small proportion of men have problems with their immune system which can lead to fertility problems. When this happens their immune system looks on their sperm as invaders and so destroys them. This problem can now be overcome, using the ICSI technique (see page 62).

Failure of sperm production

In some instances sperm production can be non-existent, even though the usual amount of semen is produced. This can be due to testicular failure – the testicles are not producing any sperm – or blockage in the fine tubing from the testicles. Surgery can be helpful in some cases but, depending on the cause, treatment may be difficult.

The testes may have become damaged as a result of an infection, the most obvious being complications as a result of mumps. Chemotherapy for cancer can cause *azoospermia* (the absence of sperm). In such cases, perhaps when a man has to have such therapy for cancer of the testicles, sperm may be collected beforehand and then frozen for use at a future date.

Impotence

Sexual problems which result in not being able to have an erection or failure to maintain an erection could be a reason for infertility.

At least half of all male impotence is due to a physical cause, such as excess alcohol, drugs that lower blood pressure and diabetes. However, other factors such as premature ejaculation can have such an adverse effect upon a man that he can become impotent.

If impotence has been present for some time, it is vital that careful psychological counselling is given. After this, various treatments can be offered. Specialists may suggest an injection and, once taught, men can inject their penis with a medicine that produces an erection. This is a great psychological boost to many impotent men and may soon return them to a natural erection-producing state. Alternatively, a surgeon can insert into the penis an inflatable rod or one made of firm but flexible material. These are expensive and not yet available on the NHS.

UNEXPLAINED INFERTILITY

In around fifteen per cent of cases of infertility, no physical cause can be found. Some specialists believe that unexplained infertility is not a diagnosis. It just means that doctors haven't found the cause.

This diagnosis can be frustrating for doctor and patient alike. For the doctor it is difficult to decide which treatment would be most appropriate and for the patient it is frustrating to be told there is a problem but nobody knows exactly what it is.

HOW COMMON IS INFERTILITY?

As many as one in six couples are thought to have problems conceiving. According to ISSUE, in Britain alone that means that there are at least two million people whose lives will be affected at some time. It is estimated that up to half a million of these people are actively seeking help at any given moment.

INVESTIGATIONS – THE FIRST PART OF TREATMENT

Investigations are a vital part of infertility treatment. Any causes for failure to conceive need to be investigated thoroughly to ensure that you receive the treatment most suited to your needs.

Provision of infertility services may vary widely in different parts of the UK. Some areas will have special fertility clinics. In other areas you may be referred to a gynaecologist or, if a sperm problem is suspected, a urologist with an interest in andrology. There are also many private fertility clinics.

TESTS FOR A MAN

Tests for a man could involve:

- semen analysis
- blood or urine tests
- X-rays or ultrasound scans
- a biopsy of the testes

Your doctor or a specialist will do an examination of the man's genitals, whether they are normal in size and in the right place (not up in the abdomen and unable to be easily moved down), and whether a varicocele, epididymal thickening or scrotal swellings are present.

Semen analysis

For a man investigations into infertility are usually straightforward and will involve semen analysis. He is asked to produce a sample of semen by masturbation and a microscopic examination of this can tell the specialist most of what he needs to know.

Although these days couples trying for a baby are advised to have sex as frequently as they wish to, when it comes to semen analysis some doctors will ask you not to have sex for two to four days before producing the sperm sample because it is thought that frequent intercourse could affect the amount of sperm in the sample and their motility. It helps in analysing the result if the specialist knows he is interpreting the best possible picture.

By counting the number of sperm swimming about within a measured amount of seminal fluid, the specialist can see whether there are enough of them, whether they are active enough, and whether the majority look normal (known as having normal morphology).

Semen is usually analysed twice at intervals of one month. This is because routine tests can be inaccurate as sperm production can be affected by other factors such as whether or not a man had an infection, such as a bout of flu, for example, three months earlier. Sometimes a factor such as a delay between the production of sperm and the time when the laboratory receives it can affect motility (movement). A sample should reach the laboratory within ninety minutes of being ejaculated as sperm motility declines quickly from then on. So don't be overanxious if your sperm needs to be analysed more than once.

Very often a semen analysis will be the first line

of investigation as it is the simplest and least intrusive of the options available.

Blood or urine tests

Blood or urine tests are carried out to check hormone levels. These can help to determine whether the part of the testes responsible for producing sperm are damaged, or whether or not there could be a blockage in the reproductive organs.

Special X-rays and scans

These can pinpoint any blockages and check whether the blood supply to the testes is efficient. The use of ultrasound assesses the prostate gland and the seminal vesicles. A vasography may be done. This is a special X-ray similar to a hysterosalpingogram (see page 40). This procedure involves checking the *vas deferens* for blockages. They can be blocked from birth or by disease.

Testicular biopsy

A tiny piece of tissue is taken from each of the testicles, under local anaesthesia, to look at sperm production.

Post-coital test

A post-coital test means exactly what it implies. A woman's cervical mucus is examined after sexual intercourse to discover what is happening to the sperm deposited in the vagina.

This procedure involves having sex a day or so before ovulation and then attending a clinic between six and eight hours later, when a sample of fluid is taken from around the cervix.

The test establishes if enough of the man's sperm are able to get through the cervical mucus and are swimming in sufficient numbers, as both these factors are essential for fertilisation to occur. Usually the mucus contains live sperm swimming around, but sometimes they are seen swimming slowly or not at all. These tests can often be repeated.

Most people undergoing infertility investigations tell me that they find this, although not uncomfortable, one of the most unpleasant procedures to go through because of its very personal nature.

TESTS FOR A WOMAN

There are also several investigative procedures that may be followed in the case of a woman. These could include:

- Temperature and hormone profiles
- Ultrasound scans
- Endometrial biopsy
- Hysterosalpingography
- Cervical examination

Temperature and hormone profiles

These may be carried out to establish whether or not a woman is ovulating properly by means of blood tests and urine tests. Blood tests can measure amounts of various hormones in the blood. For example, a blood test can reveal whether or not there are high levels of progesterone in the blood which suggests that ovulation is occurring. Urine tests can also measure amounts of hormones.

You may be asked to keep temperature charts for three to six months. Taking your temperature every day will establish if you are ovulating (see also page 19).

Ultrasound scans

Sometimes ultrasound scanning of the ovaries is carried out, usually between day seven and fourteen of a woman's cycle to confirm if an egg is being produced in the right way and then released. An ultrasound scan can also be used to check the shape of the uterus.

Endometrial biopsy

Endometrial biopsy may be done where a tiny sample of womb lining (endometrium) is checked to see if it has responded to hormonal changes. That is to see whether the lining's stage of development is in phase with the woman's hormonal cycle and is free from infection.

Hysterosalpingography

Other tests can be carried out to examine Fallopian tubes and to check tubal patency. One such test is called a hysterosalpingography. This is a type of special X-ray in which a dye is passed through the cervix, the womb and up into the Fallopian tubes to see if there are any blockages, or to assess the size and shape of the womb. This is usually done without a general anaesthetic and can feel rather uncomfortable. A hysteroscopy is another form of telescopic examination to look at the womb cavity. The hysteroscope, a narrow tube, is inserted through the cervix.

Cervical examination

When a woman has a history of miscarriage, the condition of the cervix may be checked to see whether it can support a full term pregnancy.

FURTHER INVESTIGATIONS AND TREATMENT

In brief there are three main approaches to the treatment of infertility: drug treatment, laparoscopy and surgery, and assisted conception.

Drug treatment

Fertility drugs are given to encourage the growth of follicles and induce ovulation. Drug treatment can also form part of *in vitro* fertilisation (IVF) treatment.

Laparoscopy and surgery

This is reserved for correcting structural causes of infertility, such as blockage to Fallopian tubes; the surgical removal of fibroids or to treat endometriosis.

Assisted conception

Broadly speaking this is when both the egg and sperm cells (known as gametes) are helped in some way to achieve fertilisation and pregnancy.

THE TREATMENT OF FEMALE INFERTILITY

DRUGS

There are many possibilities in this form of treatment, depending on a woman's particular problem. Problems with cervical mucus often lead to a treatment which involves the administering of small doses of oestrogen to improve the quality of the mucus. Drugs can also be used to stimulate ovulation, and are used when a woman isn't producing her monthly eggs.

There are two main types of drug. The first – and most frequently used – stimulates the 'resting' pituitary gland which, in turn, produces its own hormone that triggers ovaries to ovulate naturally. Less commonly, when a woman's pituitary gland cannot be stimulated, she may be prescribed the pituitary hormones called gonadotrophins. These directly stimulate the ovary to produce eggs.

An example of a drug commonly used when women have an ovulation problem is clomiphene (Clomid). This is given for the treatment of ovulatory failure when other causes have been ruled out. What clomiphene does is to stimulate a small gland at the base of the brain called the pituitary gland. This then puts out hormones, called pituitary gonadotrophins, which will stimulate a woman's ovaries, in particular, the development of the ova (eggs). It also stimulates those parts of the ovary responsible for putting out other hormones after the egg has been released, which are essential for a pregnancy to start.

The success or otherwise of this treatment can be measured by testing the woman's urine. This shows whether there is an increase in the output of gonadotrophins, indicating that the pituitary is working properly, and a corresponding increase in oestrogen to show that the ovaries are functioning normally.

The drug is given daily for five days. This treatment tends to be a short-term remedy as most patients will ovulate following three courses.

When neither the pituitary nor the ovary are able to be stimulated in this way, the condition is known as primary pituitary or primary ovarian failure. In these cases clomiphene is not then effective.

There are more specialist drugs – some of which will be used in IVF treatment to stimulate egg production – which are used to help a woman's body produce an ovum and increase the prospects of pregnancy. If you are going to have hormone drug treatment, do discuss the drugs that will be used and ask about the possible side-effects, such as hot flushes or the rarer hyperstimulation (when ovaries react too strongly to the drug) and the risks of multiple pregnancy.

A recent television programme highlighted the risks associated with drug treatment for infertility and the emotional, physical and financial burdens placed on couples who may have triplets, quads or even quins as a consequence.

Babies born as a result of multiple pregnancy are more likely to be premature and to have serious health problems. Even if the children are born healthy, the impact on the parents' ability to cope both mentally and financially is huge. In some instances when a woman has a multiple pregnancy, the couple face the dilemma of going through with the pregnancy, terminating it completely or undergoing a controversial operation called selective embryo reduction, in which embryos to be aborted are injected with potassium chloride. The programme pointed out the need for careful monitoring of egg production by blood oestrogen tests, and the use of ultrasound scanning to minimise the risks of multiple pregnancy.

SURGERY

Treatment of blocked Fallopian tubes involves surgery using a laparoscope. This helps about a third of women who have damaged Fallopian tubes.

A laparoscopy is an internal examination of the abdomen and pelvis undertaken by the surgeon through a laparoscope – a tube that is inserted into the abdomen through a tiny incision. Usually done under general anaesthetic, an inert gas such as carbon dioxide is pumped into the abdomen to blow it up so the organs can be more easily separated. A light is shone down the laparoscope and small cutting or cauterising implements can be manipulated through it.

Laparoscopy is an enormous advance, pioneered in this country by gynaecologists and now widely used by other surgeons. It enables the doctor to look at the Fallopian tubes and the outside of the womb, as well as the ovaries, to get a much clearer picture of what could be causing fertility problems. And, thanks to its existence, the patient can now be out of hospital in a day or two and back at work often within a week or two.

The success of tubal surgery depends on the site and degree of tubal damage or malformity and the extent of scarring. When tubes are badly damaged IVF is probably a better option. Some women will want to opt for IVF as their first type of treatment if they don't want tubal surgery.

ASSISTED CONCEPTION: *IN VITRO* FERTILISATION (IVF)

IVF or *in vitro* fertilisation may seem to some like a new technique, but in fact it has now been practised since 1978 when Robert Edwards and Patrick Steptoe had the great success with the birth of the first test tube baby Louise Brown. In the last six years alone many thousands of babies have been born in Britain as a result of IVF treatment. According to the International Health Foundation one in a hundred of all babies born in the Netherlands are conceived by *in vitro* fertilisation.

IVF, which simply means fertilisation outside the body, is not the answer to every fertility problem, and it is important that people seeking help with conception should understand this from the outset. There is no hard guarantee that if you pursue this course of treatment you will end up with a baby. You need to be prepared for what you are letting yourself in for.

IVF is used for women with tubal abnormalities and infertility due to certain hormonal causes. It can help in some cases when couples experience unexplained infertility and for women with hostile cervical mucus (which rejects sperm) or endometriosis (see page 26). IVF can also be carried out on women whose infertility is mainly due to male factors. Donor sperm can also be used, as can donated eggs (see page 51) and IVF is used with the new micromanipulation techniques (see page 61).

Basically IVF allows an egg to be introduced into a woman's womb. The specialist takes a woman's eggs and mixes them with her partner's, or a donor's, sperm, then returns them two or three days after fertilisation to the womb. Hopefully, nature takes over and goes on to form and nurture a baby.

Normally IVF clinics will administer hormonal drugs to the patient which will stimulate the maturation of several eggs in one monthly cycle and these will be collected for use in treatment. Collecting several eggs at one time means that two or three embryos can be replaced, thereby increasing the chances of pregnancy in one treatment cycle. It also avoids the need for extra surgery, since egg collection involves an operation under a general anaesthetic or now, increasingly commonly, a mild sedative which has made it a quick and relatively straightforward procedure. Some clinics do not stimulate the ovaries, but collect the egg that is produced naturally. This is referred to as Natural Cycle IVF.

Drugs that can be used in IVF treatment are:

• *Buserelin* (Suprefact), a hormone suppressant which may be administered in the form of a nasal spray or daily injection. This drug damps down the action of the pituitary gland which is the gland controlling ovary stimulation. The ovaries can consequently be stimulated artificially.
• *HMG Human Menopausal Gonadotrophin* (Pergonal, Humegon) stimulates the development of egg follicles in order to increase the number of oocytes available for collection.

- *FSH Follicle Stimulating Hormone* (Metrodin)
- *Clomiphene Citrate* (Serophene) is sometimes given in combination with gonadotrophins to induce multiple follicular maturation – and hence to increase the ova production.
- *HCG Human Chorionic Gonadotrophin* (Gonadotraphon LH, Pregnyl or Profasi) is administered by injection about thirty-six hours before egg collection, either by laparoscopy or ultrasound-guided aspiration (see page 48). It helps to ripen the eggs within the follicles.

Before this final injection there will be ultrasound scanning to establish how many eggs are developing on the ovaries. The scanning will show the number of follicles developing and their size. If a woman has over-responded to the drugs and too many eggs have been produced, the injection may be cancelled and the treatment cycle abandoned. Checks like this help to minimise the risks of ovarian hyperstimulation syndrome, which can cause fluid-filled cysts appearing on the ovaries.

Some of these drugs can be taken by mouth but most have to be given by injection. Clinics may give the daily injections themselves or they may arrange for a GP or local hospital to give them. The last injection has to be carefully timed so that eggs to be collected are mature, but will not have been released by the ovary. It might have to be given late at night and this could cause some inconvenience. Sometimes training can be given so that the injections can be self-administered or administered by a partner. Many women undergoing IVF find this helpful.

Taking drugs containing hormones is not without its drawbacks. Some women find they suffer certain unpleasant side-effects, such as hot flushes, depression, headaches, sometimes nausea, vomiting, diarrhoea, dizziness, or not being able to sleep properly at night. Sometimes a woman can 'over-react' to these drugs, known as hyperstimulation. So if you are receiving drug treatment as part of a course of IVF, do ask your doctor about side-effects you might experience and contact your clinic if you experience any unexpectedly unpleasant symptoms.

Egg collection is a routine part of IVF (unless donated eggs are being used). The most common way of collecting them is by using an ultrasound-guided needle to 'aspirate', or remove, the eggs. This involves the insertion of a very fine hollow needle through the vagina in order to remove the eggs. Women find that this can be quite unpleasant and uncomfortable. It is helpful if painkillers are taken before egg collection is carried out.

Another way of collecting eggs is by laparoscopy (see page 44).

Shortly before egg collection a sperm sample will be required from your partner. The most motile sperm are selected and are mixed with the egg or eggs and incubated overnight. If fertilisation has occurred the embryos will be replaced or they can be stored for use at a later date.

IVF treatment is carefully controlled by the Human Fertilisation and Embryology Authority (HFEA). According to their guidelines, up to three embryos can be transferred into the patient's womb. This is done using a fine catheter (plastic tube). More than one embryo is usually transferred to allow a greater likelihood of pregnancy.

Depending on the levels of hormones in your

blood and the type of drugs you will already have been prescribed, you may have to have hormone injections to stop your ovaries beginning another cycle. There then follows a two-week wait to see whether treatment has been successful and the embryo has implanted in the uterus wall.

I am often asked about the success rate of IVF. In an efficient clinic, the chances of getting pregnant from any IVF attempt are one in five, which is not that different from the chance of natural conception. Some studies show that the chance of pregnancy from one IVF treatment cycle is comparable, and in some instances might be slightly better than a natural cycle. An ordinarily fertile couple having regular unprotected sexual intercourse has a one in five to one in four chance of conception. However, success rates vary from one centre to another. The chance of success is also an individual factor dependent on the woman's age (success rates fall after the age of thirty-eight), your own particular cause of infertility and the couple's previous history of infertility treatment. Certainly statistics show that the more treatment cycles you have the more chance you have of getting pregnant – although that is cold comfort for those who are struggling financially to fund treatment from their own incomes or savings. According to one study reported in the *British Medical Journal* the overall 'cumulative probability of pregnancy' after six cycles of IVF treatment is eighty-two per cent. This means that eighty-two of a hundred women starting out on IVF treatment programmes will be pregnant by the time the sixth successive treatment cycle is reached.

On another positive note, there are continual advances in infertility treatment, which is evolving all the time. Research into IVF is also going on constantly in the hope of 'perfecting' the technique. Research has recently revealed that special cells, called granulosa cells or 'nurse' cells, surround eggs developing in the ovary which help it to mature. Researchers have identified a link between an enzyme produced by these cells and the failure of embryos to implant in the uterus. It is hoped that testing for this enzyme would help to identify cycles in which embryos would not implant, thus avoiding unnecessary financial cost, treatment and anxiety.

GIFT

GIFT, or gamete intrafallopian transfer, is a similar technique to IVF. In this case, the eggs collected from the ovary are switched back to the Fallopian tube, along with a small sample of sperm almost immediately after collection. The difference between the techniques is mainly that fertilisation in GIFT occurs in the natural environment of the Fallopian tube. In 'natural' conception, the egg has to enter the Fallopian tube and so GIFT may help women with unexplained infertility, in whom this stage in their cycle may be impaired. Up to three eggs will be transferred during each cycle. This treatment carries with it a slight risk of an ectopic pregnancy.

ZIFT

Zygote intrafallopian transfer (ZIFT) combines the techniques of IVF and GIFT. Zygote is the name for an early stage embryo and in ZIFT the first stages of fertilisation are allowed to take place in the laboratory before being transferred to the Fallopian tube.

EGG DONATION

Egg donation is sometimes needed if a young woman has a premature menopause and is no longer producing eggs, or in the case of a woman whose own eggs have failed to fertilise, or to avoid the passing on of a genetic disorder. NEEDS, the National Egg and Embryo Donation Society, points out that there is an ever increasing number of infertile women or those carrying a genetic disorder who need treatment by IVF. This may be by using either donated eggs or embryos to overcome their childlessness or to prevent the birth of a child afflicted by a debilitating genetic disease such as cystic fibrosis.

A recent survey has shown that just under 2,000 women in the UK need treatment with donated eggs and/or embryos. About half the units providing treatment by IVF in the UK already offer treatment using donated eggs and a large proportion use donated embryos.

The major limiting factor is the shortage of suitable egg donors. The provision of such treatment is regulated by the Human Fertilisation and Embryology Authority (HFEA) and the authority has indicated that gametes for the treatment of others should not be taken from female donors over the age of thirty-five unless there are exceptional reasons.

When eggs are collected from a fertile woman, and not obtained as a result of another woman's IVF treatment, the two women involved in this type of fertilisation process must both undergo treatment. For a woman to get pregnant by egg donation, the treatment process is similar apart from the need for egg collection. For the woman donating the eggs, the same drug administration and egg collection is carried out as if she were an IVF patient, while the recipient is given the two principal female hormones – oestrogen and progesterone – to mimic a normal 'pregnant' cycle. Once the eggs are collected from the donor, they are fertilised with a prepared sperm sample from the recipient's partner. Up to three embryos are transferred to the uterus two or three days after fertilisation; the rest are usually stored for use at a subsequent date.

Christine, a thirty-four-year-old industrial chemist, found that after being off the Pill for a year at the age of twenty-six and having regular unprotected sex, she was not pregnant. However, she has become pregnant after IVF treatment and believes she was fortunate that she and her husband decided not to join a three-year NHS waiting list and were not too intimidated to try private treatment.

> When I didn't get pregnant after a year I wondered whether it was because I was worrying too much. My doctor told us it was early days and a year was not a particularly long time, but nevertheless she referred us to a fertility clinic – although we waited months for the appointment. It was quite a tense time for us. I waited every month and hoped I would be pregnant. Then my period would arrive and I'd know I wasn't.
>
> Everybody around you is getting pregnant and there seems to be a lot of pressure on you to do the same. People would comment that we had been married for so long, when were we going to start a family? That would be so hurtful.

Once Christine began routine tests she felt a little more positive because at least she felt she was taking action to sort out whatever problem there was. Extensive tests revealed nothing. This added to Christine's frustration and disappointment.

> I was in agony after a laparoscopy and I was hoping that something would have been found. But I was told a reason couldn't be found. Everything was fine. My tubes were all right. I seemed to be ovulating and a problem couldn't be found. I felt very frustrated. At least if somebody gives you an answer you can face it and then deal with it. Not knowing is terrible. I was told that I could go on the NHS list for IVF but we would be looking at a three-year waiting list. There was also no guarantee I would be treated because their programme treated female infertility problems and as far as they were concerned they couldn't find one with me. So I could wait three years and then I might get refused.

The lack of a positive option spurred Christine into finding out about other avenues of treatment. She did not want to wait any longer, particularly as a cause for her infertility could not be found, so she decided to go private. She and her husband went through another round of tests and then two attempts at IVF before finally having a much-longed-for son.

> I was apprehensive because I didn't know what was going to happen. I hadn't told anyone at work, in case it failed. There were

some aspects of treatment my husband and I didn't talk to each other about while it was happening. Now we laugh about them. The classic was when my husband had to give a sperm sample. He was taken into this room and given a little tub and a dirty magazine. He was so embarrassed. That was something we didn't talk about while we were going through it.

I don't think I coped too badly with the treatment. You have to have lots of injections and ultrasound, but you have to think all the while that this could work. You have to be positive. I was warned about the possible risks of multiple pregnancy and three is a frightening thought.

My husband was very much in awe of treatment, possibly because he wasn't needed until it was time for me to have eggs collected. I don't think I had too bad a time with the side-effects of the egg-stimulating drugs. I really believed in the treatment. At the first attempt I had two embryos put back. I found that upsetting after all the treatment and time it had taken to find out that only two were suitable. I was still very positive, however, that I was pregnant.

When the first attempt failed Christine was devastated. She and her husband decided to leave treatment for a year. They moved house and tried to focus on other things. By the time they decided to try for IVF again, they met unexpected opposition which made them extremely angry.

As we'd moved house, we'd changed GP. Our doctor did not agree with IVF – probably because I don't think he knew very much about it. The first time we had treatment we were able to get the drugs we needed on the National Health. This doctor refused so we had to pay for them ourselves. We never went to see him again after that. We had to find another £1500 for the drugs. It made me really angry. I'd been working for years and paying National Insurance and for what?

When the second attempt worked I was just shocked. I was crying and shaking. I couldn't believe it. I was very nervous throughout my pregnancy. I'd go to the doctor with all sorts of pains. My doctor reassured me that I was pregnant, and no different from any woman who was pregnant. Once I got past twelve to fourteen weeks I began to feel slightly more relaxed.

Now I have a child I do look on him as very special because of what we went through. I think other IVF parents feel the same way.

Some people do have very narrow views of infertility and IVF which stem from ignorance. It's more often older people who are prejudiced. I remember one woman remarking in a very surprised voice about how he was a normal baby. I wondered what on earth she expected him to look like.

THE TREATMENT OF MALE INFERTILITY

Treatment of male infertility is a more difficult area. Surgery may help in a few cases and drugs have sometimes been used with limited success. For example, steroids may be used in cases of sperm antibodies or hormone drugs to improve sperm production. Where there is definite evidence of a local infection antibiotics to clear up the infection may assist sperm counts, but in the main other treatments are used.

ARTIFICIAL INSEMINATION

Artificial insemination is also known as AID (artificial insemination by donor, who remains anonymous) or AIH (artificial insemination by husband) or AIP (artificial insemination by partner). Around 3,000 couples try donor insemination each year in the UK.

Up until very recently donor insemination was the most common option for male infertility. It could well be, though, that following recent advances in the treatment of male infertility, such as the micromanipulation techniques we talk about below (see page 61), the demand for donor insemination will not be so great, although some doctors believe that it is still the simplest and most cost-effective treatment for most cases of male infertility. It really depends upon the feelings and wishes of both partners and how important they see the transfer of the genes of the male partner – i.e., the legal father-to-be – in the conception and characteristics of their future child.

The introduction of the Human Fertilisation and Embryology Act in 1990 means there are strict controls for the screening of donors. These involve investigation of their family medical history and the quarantining of semen samples by freezing in liquid nitrogen. This quarantine period prevents the possibility of transferring the HIV virus.

Donor insemination may be offered if there are fertility problems with the male partner, but it can also be offered when a man carries an inherited disease.

It may appear a simple process, but don't be misled into thinking that it will be a one-off experience. You may need between five and ten treatments before getting pregnant. Sperm will be deposited at the cervix (neck of the womb) close to the time of ovulation, 'mimicking', if you like, the way sperm is deposited in normal sexual intercourse. This means that the sperm then have to swim through the usual cervical mucus.

Clinics vary in their approach to insemination and how the best time for insemination is decided upon. Sometimes a woman will monitor her own ovulation time. Other clinics prefer a series of hormone tests to be carried out or a woman may take drugs to control her menstrual cycle.

Intra-uterine Insemination (IUI)
Intra-uterine insemination means that specially prepared sperm are placed directly into the womb, using a fine tube placed through the cervix. This can be carried out with the most motile of donor sperm or all of the partner's sperm, and is timed to

coincide with ovulation. It can also be performed with or without ovarian stimulation.

Sperm for intra-uterine insemination are prepared germfree, either by a washing technique, or by using a sperm separation method to isolate for use those sperm that are the most motile (active). The prepared solution of sperm is drawn into a sterile catheter and introduced into the uterus directly through the neck of the womb.

It seems that IUI is more successful than vaginal insemination, where sperm is placed by syringe into the vagina. However, it does depend on healthy Fallopian tubes, and does need large numbers of healthy sperm. In its favour, the IUI procedure does have the possible advantage of allowing sperm to pass through cervical mucus. This will overcome a known problem of hostile cervical mucus, for example, when the mucus is adversely reacting with the sperm and preventing their natural passage into the womb.

Amanda, a twenty-nine-year-old analyst, who has polycystic ovaries, and her husband Gavin, a thirty-one-year-old sales and marketing executive, who has sperm antibodies, have had successful IUI. They now have a baby son. They believe that if you are going to have private treatment it's important to choose a consultant you feel comfortable with and one who has a positive attitude to your case. Amanda and Gavin had three attempts at IUI. Amanda found the treatment quite clinical, and more distressing for her than Gavin, who had to produce sperm specimens on demand.

> Having to do it for the set appointment and I'd be wanting to say 'Come on, hurry up'. But you can't say that or then it would not

work at all. That was a strain. I'd rush it to hospital. I'd wait an hour for the sperm to be prepared. Treatment felt like having a smear test, but a bit more uncomfortable. You have to lie flat for twenty minutes. My consultant was brilliant. He would sit there and talk to me.

During that time I would pray that it would work. You spend two weeks of the month being positive. I'd go to hospital every day for injections and scans. Then when it doesn't work you're down. You go from really optimistic to really pessimistic.

Amanda was so overjoyed about being pregnant on the third attempt she didn't even tell anyone for a whole day until she had a second positive pregnancy test. While Amanda had often wondered whether she would ever become a mother, Gavin was fairly optimistic that something would be sorted out.

What was very important to my feelings was that before all this happened Amanda had had a miscarriage. Because I knew we had been able to have a conception, it made it easier to be optimistic that one day we would have a child.

It's curious, but in a sense I was relieved when it was discovered that I had a problem as well. By this time Amanda was very churned up about the whole thing. She had a sense of inadequacy. So for there to be something wrong with me, and for us to share it, was a relief. It made me feel as if we were in it together.

I remember being surprised at the way I felt. I thought I was supposed to feel desperately inadequate about it all. What helped was that I had sperm antibodies, and as my condition is quite unusual it almost made me feel special. I feared us not being able to have a child and us adopting. I think not being able to have a child of our own would have upset me. From my point of view there was the need to re-create myself and to have the family continuing on. The sense that that's what generations past had done, so that's what I should do.

At one stage, however, when Amanda was becoming more and more distressed about not becoming pregnant Gavin wondered what the outcome would be.

I felt that somewhere along the line a toll would be taken on our relationship. I wondered what would happen if we didn't solve something. I still felt it would work at some point because we had identified the problems. I was more scared of any pregnancy not lasting. There was also a point when the treatment was taking its toll on Amanda and there were tears every month on the appointed day. I tried to be as understanding as possible, but you run out of words of comfort. Amanda was under such strain and I felt a slight sense of guilt that I was able to take it in my stride.

MICROMANIPULATION TECHNIQUES

The different techniques of micro-assisted fertilisation (MAF) all involve the use of extremely powerful microscopes and micromanipulators which hold an egg and penetrate it with a needle seven or more times smaller than a human hair.

Partial zona dissection (PZD)
Partial zona dissection (PZD) involves making a hole in the outer layer (zona) of a single human egg, to facilitate penetration and fertilisation by the sperm cells.

Sub-zona insemination (SUZI)
Sub-zona insemination (SUZI) takes PZD a stage further and puts sperm in direct contact with an egg by using a micro-needle. It actually positions a few individual sperm cells, or even only one, just beneath the outer 'shell' of the egg, so they only have to pass into the cytoplasm – the tissue of the cell but not its gene centre – of the egg to achieve fertilisation. The sperm will then be best able to reach the centre of the cell, where its own genes, from the man, can join with the genes of the ovary, from the woman.

Computer image sperm selection (CISS)
CISS is another significant advance being pioneered by British scientists at Nottingham University Research and Treatment Unit in Reproduction (NURTURE). By using a special type of scanner called a real time computer imaging system, which was originally developed to monitor traffic flow, the scientists have been able to

pick out fertile sperm which can then be injected into the egg. It used to be thought that the sperm most likely to fertilise an egg was the one that was the fastest swimmer but, interestingly, researchers have now discovered that it is the sperm which moves with extra thrashing actions to enable it to get through the egg's barrier that has the most chance of success. CISS selects the potentially most viable sperm and can be used with the SUZI or ICSI techniques to boost chances of successful conception.

Micro-epididymal sperm aspiration (MESA)
Yet another advance is micro-epididymal sperm aspiration (MESA). This is a technique originally developed in the USA which removes a small specimen of semen from the epididymis – the tubes that carry sperm from where they are produced in the testes to their storage site and eventually to the outside. It is a microscopical technique which uses cells aspirated (sucked) from the epididymis for MAF (or IVF if there are adequate sperm). The experimental success of MESA suggests that in men who are azoospermic (contain no sperm in their semen) it is now possible to obtain sperm from the epididymis in order to fertilise their partner's eggs.

Intra-cytoplasmic sperm injection (ICSI)
This is another micro-assisted fertilisation technique – probably the latest and most exciting – which recently received a great deal of publicity. A breakthrough in the treatment of male infertility, ICSI is a micromanipulation technique of intra-

cytoplasmic sperm injection which appears to have ousted the other techniques of microfertilisation. The work pioneered by the Brussels Free University certainly appears remarkable and offers great hope for the treatment of male infertility. Some experts have compared ICSI in the treatment of male infertility to the impact IVF had as a treatment for female infertility in 1978. Others are more cautious about raising false hopes and point out that this treatment is complex and expensive – but, even so, admit that it offers a great deal of promise for the future.

The new treatment means that men with poor quality sperm can father their own genetic child and offers hope when fertilisation has failed in conventional IVF because sperm has been unable to penetrate the egg. It also means that provided the male partner has some sperm somewhere in the male reproductive tract and the couple are prepared to persist with IVF, more couples than ever before will be able to have their own genetic babies.

Sperm heads are 5 microns (five millionth of a metre) across and an egg is 120–125 microns. ICSI is a technique which injects a single human sperm cell through the outer layer (*zona pellucida*) and right into the cytoplasm of the egg. The technique involves using a needle ten times finer than a human hair. It is really only the living genes in the centre, or nucleus, of the sperm cell, the complex chemical called DNA, which is needed to start a baby. Consequently, if the man's sperm are immotile, or have antibodies on their surface, it makes no difference to the likelihood of success. With the exception of one particularly rare sperm deformation, it can be said that virtually all of the male problems of infertility can be overcome using ICSI.

Fortunately, the success rate for fertilisation using this technique is remarkably high (nearly sixty per cent). Of these fertilised eggs, nine out of ten become successful embryos, able to be used for insertion into a woman. Almost one in five women fertilised in this way delivered a healthy baby. These statistics compare more than favourably with the natural process of trying to conceive by normal intercourse. The figures are even more re-markable when one considers that this success rate is based on couples with long-term infertility prob-lems, who may have been totally unable to achieve conception by normal means. The men involved may have had few if any sperm in their ejaculation and any sperm ejaculated may have been totally immobile.

To reiterate, it is thought that this process offers about a one in four chance of success with each attempt. Results so far seem better than standard IVF results. And, although a new process, many of the treatment centres in the UK are already offer-ing this fertilisation technique.

As ever with new techniques, time will tell if the early promise of ICSI lives up to the expectations. Responsible scientists are always a little cautious with any new technique, and they are now waiting and watching to see what, if any, problems arise.

ALTERNATIVE TREATMENTS

Most practitioners of unconventional therapies prefer the use of the term 'complementary' medicine rather than 'alternative' because they feel their treatment should work side by side with more conventional methods. No responsible alternative practitioner would suggest that they have the cure for all human ills. On the other hand, a person will sometimes be helped by an alternative practitioner after his or her many symptoms have been fully investigated and no abnormality other than the symptoms themselves has been discovered. If traditional medicine is not helping, you have nothing to lose by talking to responsible alternative practitioners. John Dickson, of ISSUE, believes that alternative therapies may not be the answer to getting pregnant but that they could help people cope with the stress of infertility treatment.

If you do try an alternative therapy, go to a practitioner who is registered with the relevant professional organisation. Also, make sure that they are insured against negligence and that you can afford their fees. And don't go if your doctor has advised against it.

So what's available? Examples are:

ACUPUNCTURE

Acupuncture has been an accepted form of treatment in China for around 5000 years and these days more and more people in the West are turning to it. Acupuncture aims to correct any disharmony within the body – to achieve a balance between Yin and Yang. An imbalance, acupuncturists say, can lead to disease. There are different traditions of acupuncture, but they all revolve around the basic principle that the body has an intricate network of linking pathways, or 'meridians', which carry our vital 'energies' through the body. These cannot be seen, but can be detected using special techniques.

During acupuncture very fine needles are inserted into several 'acupoints' according to the problem being treated. By inserting needles or by using pressure, the correct flow and balance of energies can be restored. One theory is that acupuncture stimulates the brain to produce endorphins, the body's natural painkillers.

HOMOEOPATHY

Homoeopathy works on the theory that less is more and that like cures like. Symptoms are treated by giving a minute dose of a substance which, if given in larger quantities to a healthy person, would actually cause those symptoms.

Even in conventional medicine this principle is sometimes used – for instance, controlled doses of radiation are given to cure cancer, which can itself be caused by too much radiation. No one has so far been able to explain exactly how homoeopathy works, however. One theory is that a form of radiation energy is released which stimulates the body's own healing mechanisms.

As homoeopathy is a holistic therapy (a therapy treating the whole person), part of the treatment process involves taking a detailed background history, and people do find that this alone can be a form of counselling. The aim is to match the remedy to the individual patient. Remedies often used in the treatment of infertility are Sepia and Carcinosin but, of course, remedies vary from person to person.

HERBAL MEDICINE

'Herbs' (which include a variety of plants, flowers and even trees) have been used for thousands of years to cure or prevent disease. Even today eighty-five per cent of the world's population is largely dependent on herbal medicine. Like homoeopathy, herbal medicine aims not just to treat a particular symptom, but to improve the overall physical and mental well-being of the patient. In herbalism it is thought important to consider the physical state of our bodies before we even try to conceive. Herbal medicines may also be used to treat irregular periods, fibroids, ovarian cysts and endometriosis among other problems.

Medicines are usually given in the form of a 'tincture' – a concentrated solution made from suitable herbs which have been soaked in water and alcohol. Sometimes the herbalist provides the actual plants from which to make an 'infusion' (similar to tea) or a 'decoction', whereby the plants are gently simmered for some time and the juices then strained off. Medicinal herbs can also be given as suppositories, ointments and poultices.

REFLEXOLOGY

The origins of reflexology can be traced back thousands of years and the technique is thought to have been used by the Ancient Egyptians. The art of foot reflexology was established in the 1930s by an American therapist called Eunice Ingham.

Reflexology works on the understanding that there are areas, called reflex points, on the feet and also on the hands, which match up with each organ, gland and structure of the body. The sole of the foot is thought to represent a map of the body. The spine's reflex point is along the inside edge of both feet which is supposed to be similar in shape to that of the spine. The four arches of the spine – cervical, thoracic, lumbar and sacral – are reflected in the four arches of the feet.

A treatment of reflexology can last around thirty to forty minutes. It is likely to involve a variety of massage techniques using the thumb and index finger in addition to a way of rotating the foot, called reflex rotation or pivot-point technique. The technique is a gentle one and many people find it quite pleasurable and relaxing. It is considered that the main benefit is its powers of relaxation, which can relieve stress and tension. It is also said to re-store balance, to improve blood supply and to encourage the unblocking of nerve impulses.

YOGA

Yoga has been practised in India for centuries as a means of maintaining mental and physical health. Do not rush into things if you start a yoga class, however; take it slowly but surely.

ALEXANDER TECHNIQUE

Another alternative therapy which could help you deal with stress efficiently is the Alexander Tech-nique. This is a gentle method aimed at relaxing muscles and improving posture by undoing bad sitting and standing habits. An Alexander Technique teacher can point out to you areas of tension which you were not even aware of, and show how you trigger off this tension at the thought of movement. He or she will instruct you on how to prevent this. Most importantly, the teacher improves your awareness of your body so that you can recognise tension before it builds to the point of causing muscle pain.

OSTEOPATHY

Osteopathy is the most orthodox of the unorthodox therapies. It believes that many diseases are due to parts of the skeleton being misplaced and should consequently be treated by gentle methods of adjustment. Osteopaths use a variety of techniques, ranging from gentle massage or stretching movements to manipulation.

CHIROPRACTIC

Chiropractic is similar to osteopathy and is based on manipulation of the spine. Chiropractors believe that most problems occur because of misalignment, or 'subluxation', of one or more of the vertebrae. They say this can irritate, pinch or cause pressure on a nerve, resulting in pain or symptoms.

Osteopathic treatment tends to include more soft-tissue techniques (various types of massage) than chiropractic, and indirect rather than direct ways of adjusting (manipulating) the affected joints. There are also many similarities in the methods used, however. Neither treatment includes any form of surgery and very rarely drugs, which greatly enhances their appeal to many people.

HOW TO DEAL WITH YOUR DOCTOR

It could be useful in the future if as soon as you decide to seek medical help you keep a file and note down the dates of appointments, what advice you were given, and the names of the doctors or specialists you saw.

Few of us like having to consult our doctor. In infertility, problems concern 'intimate' parts of our bodies and our private life. I wish I could convince everyone that there is no need for embarrassment. Your doctor has dealt with infertility before and examining any part of the male or female body is just part of the day's work. Research has shown that fertility problems are one of the most common reasons for patients visiting the surgery.

Your first line of action should be a visit to your GP. Don't be embarrassed about what your doctor may want to know. The GP may ask questions about:

- Your age and what you do for a living
- What sort of contraception you have previously used
- Your menstrual cycle and whether you might have had problems in the past – infrequent periods are those which are more than forty-two days apart
- Whether you have had any previous pregnancies
- How often you and your partner make love and if you have any sexual problems

- Whether or not you smoke, drink alcohol or take illegal drugs
- Whether or not you are suffering from stress
- If the male partner has had any genito-urinary infections
- The general health of both families.

In some cases the GP may advise you to carry on trying for a while longer or he or she may advise further investigations straight away, particularly if:

- You have been trying to get pregnant for more than a year
- The female partner is over thirty years of age
- You have already had a miscarriage
- Your medical history means that you've had problems in the past – pelvic infection in a woman, for example, or a scrotal injury in a man
- It is also important to try to remember or note any pyrexial illnesses – illnesses during which you've had a raised temperature – in the previous six months.

Hopefully you will meet with a sensitive and sympathetic approach, which will make facing up to and dealing with any problems that much more acceptable. If you're not happy with your GP, be prepared to change doctor.

No matter how rushed your doctor, or hospital specialist, may seem, it is still important for you to make the most of the time you've got with him or her. So there is absolutely no harm in preparing yourself mentally for a visit. It helps many people to write down a list of questions, or a list of things they don't understand and would like explained in more detail or more simply. I know it may be difficult, but don't be intimidated or anxious about asking questions.

If you don't understand what you're being told, make sure your doctor realises this and ask for it to be explained more slowly, or more simply. You needn't feel embarrassed or stupid. You certainly won't be the first person they've seen who's had difficulty grasping all the facts. And you won't be the last. Don't be afraid to write down any answers you are given either. It is not unusual for someone seeing a doctor to remember only about a third of what they've been told.

If you are worried about something in particular, make sure you ask questions about it. There is nothing worse than anxiety that stems from ignorance. Tell your doctor of any secret fears you have as he or she can then usually reassure you and prevent unnecessary worry. Make sure you understand why a certain avenue of treatment is being suggested for you. And if you have to wait for an appointment to see a specialist, do ring secretaries and appointment clerks to see if there are any cancellations.

Remember to ask about the possible side-effects and risks of any treatment and the risks of multiple pregnancy if that is appropriate.

Bear in mind that not all health authorities fund infertility treatments. I receive many letters from anxious couples who have heard that their local health authority is giving IVF a low priority. This is because the priority given to non-emergency treatments can now be determined by the health authorities (now called purchasing authorities). Some of them allow IVF treatment on the NHS, but restrict the attempts to three. And as the chance of getting pregnant from any IVF attempt is one in five, if a couple is unlucky a pregnancy might not occur after three attempts. Whether a couple can get more IVF treatment on the NHS is something they will have to put to their health authority, their local Community Health Council (the official watchdog body) and/or their local MP.

You should be aware that if you need treatment such as ICSI, which is not available in your region, you can apply for it at a centre elsewhere under an NHS system known as extra-contractual referral (ECR). Of course this does not guarantee treatment, but each authority does have a certain amount of cash available for out-of-area referrals. If you are having problems getting permission for the funds to flow, write to the chairman of your local health authority. You will find the telephone number under NHS in the local telephone directory. You could also write to the director of public health of the authority or the ECR manager, if there is one.

Readers may like to join the National Infertility Awareness Campaign which was organised to create more awareness of infertility and to convince health ministers and officials that more modern and cost-effective investigation and treatment should be offered routinely by district health authorities and regional health boards in preference to older treatments which have lower success rates. The Campaign's other objectives are to achieve uniform provision and a full range of infertility investigation and treatments throughout the country. For an information pack ring Freephone 0800 716345.

TURNING TO THE PRIVATE SECTOR

Seemingly endless waiting lists and the limited availability of infertility treatment drive many towards private medicine, even when they can hardly afford it. If you are thinking about turning to the private sector for help, remember that you are paying not for a baby but for a chance of a baby. It carries no guarantee.

Do not be intimidated about asking to see your particular clinic's result tables for any treatment you may be about to embark on. The same advice applies to NHS clinics as well. When choosing a clinic think about how all aspects of treatment are going to affect you, not just the success rates. Success rates in themselves could be misleading anyway because they depend on a variety of factors, not least the age of the patients being treated and the reasons for their fertility problems.

Things you should think about include the cost and exactly what that cost covers, the clinic's waiting list length, how much travelling you might have to do and how many times you might have to attend. Ask exactly what services are available, whether or not the clinic specialises, are there any age restrictions and so on. A comprehensive leaflet called *Treatment Clinic: Questions to Ask* is available from the Human Fertilisation and Embryology Authority (see page 102).

Before offering treatment, clinics are obliged to consider the welfare of any resulting child, together with any other child who could be affected by the birth.

And a last word of advice: if you become pregnant do inform the medical staff involved in your case.

INFERTILITY AND EMOTIONS

Most people have a deep and instinctive desire to have children. When that instinct is not fulfilled, the infertile couple have a constant and frustrating battle with their emotions as they try to cope.

People have told me that infertility makes you grieve in a similar way to bereavement. Some say it is harder to grieve for children who never existed rather than being able to focus your grief on a person who has. Bereavement also inspires more understanding as it is something everyone will have to face at some time. People with infertility problems struggle to hide their emotions, so those around them cannot understand what they are going through. They feel guilty about some of their feelings – and they feel angry too. Anger can be turned against the other partner – the one to 'blame', or the one who insisted that you go to the doctor in the first place – or it can be turned inwards.

Other emotions include anxiety – while waiting to see if a treatment has worked; guilt – about things that have happened in the past that make people think it's all their own fault; isolation – they feel they are the only ones with this problem, particularly as infertility is still a subject not everyone can discuss openly; frustration – with the health service or at being expected to perform sexually on demand; and in many cases depression, and feelings of pointlessness. Loss of self-esteem is also common, as is a feeling of failure and inadequacy.

That sense of failure and inadequacy can also have a knock-on effect on other areas of a person's life, especially if all is not going well at work. Unfortunately, many people are striving to make their mark at work or further their careers at around the same age as they are having to deal with fertility problems. Sexual difficulties also develop. It is not surprising if a man feels he has to perform 'to order', that the requirement to do so – an erection – is less likely to occur spontaneously, causing further distress to what in any case may be, by now, a tense relationship.

If either partner has a particularly anxious or depressive tendency, the strain of infertility can tip the balance so that they will need support, if not treatment, for anxiety and depression as well.

ISSUE's John Dickson believes the emotional side of infertility is very important.

> Everybody comes to us for information but what they also need is support and counselling. Infertility treatment offers a hard road to follow even if you do succeed. If you are three or four years infertile you can't undo the hurt that was done to you, the effect it has on your sexuality and that kind of thing. This is very seldom dealt with. People can be bruised and very hurt for years afterwards by the things others said to them or by the way their parents reacted.
>
> When you are infertile, something precious has been stripped away from you. It is something everybody takes for granted. If you are suddenly very ill you see how precious life is. But most people want to have children and when you can't and you stare

down that black hole of not having any babies at all, it is like facing death. Indeed, what you are facing is your own genetic death. If you can face this you can learn a lot about yourself and you can have a strengthened marriage because of it.

Dealing with their emotions and talking about how they feel can be healing for many people, yet in general it seems that men cannot find this release to the same extent as women.

Wendy, who is a volunteer on CHILD's Linkline, a twenty-four-hour helpline, believes that although infertility itself is not new, the latest treatments are throwing up a new set of taboos and moral issues which some people can talk about but others cannot.

In a way infertility is a new subject. Whereas once if you could not have children that was that, now medical advances mean that there are a whole new set of problems and a new set of taboos. Some people are very open about their feelings, but some women ring up and their partners don't even know about their infertility. Sometimes, once people have got a child, say by IVF, they want nothing more to do with infertility. They don't want to be involved in anything to do with it and behave as if it never happened.

Wendy believes men have more difficulty than women in 'talking babies'.

Men seem to think that male infertility is tied up with virility, which is nonsense. The man who fires blanks, as it were, just does not want this known. In my experience with Linkline I would say that ninety-nine per cent of callers are female. Women want information, but they also want to talk about how upset they are and they will talk about their feelings. Men make up about one per cent of calls and about ninety per cent of them want information about a particular situation. I have only ever had two men ring me up to say that infertility problems were affecting their relationship and who wanted to talk about how they felt.

Infertility poses a different set of problems for a man to deal with and most find it is frightening, threatening and forces them to question their value in life. But all too often men are not offered medical advice or counselling – and neither do they always seek it. They often deny the problem exists.

Tracy, a twenty-nine-year-old nurse, who is currently having intra-uterine insemination (IUI), believes that sometimes the attitudes of people, including members of the medical profession, do not help men face up to problems easily.

My husband and I tend not to talk about our infertility problems really. I'm not sure whether it's a conscious decision or not. I don't know whether it's a form of self-defence, but I always think the worst and that it's not going to happen. I try to protect my feelings and I try to protect my husband's feelings. He has a low sperm count and I have endometriosis. If there has to be something wrong with either of us, I would rather it was just me because I can cope better than he can. There's so much stigma attached to male infertility problems.

We haven't had much help at coping with our problems. I've found the more junior doctors are much more approachable. I've felt able to question them because there are issues you want to ask about. In all the rush in and out, it's so impersonal yet it's such an important issue to you, sometimes medical staff don't seem to be aware of the emotional turmoil you're going through.

My husband has a low sperm count problem, yet he's never been seen by anybody, never been examined and nobody has suggested it either. Nobody has ever discussed it with him. We don't know if any tests can be done or even why he has the problem. He feels very isolated and confused.

Infertility forces people to confront all sorts of issues. The thought of a life without children can be too much to bear. Some people believe that a life without children is not richer or poorer than life for those who have children, it is simply different.

Coming to terms with the way you feel can be a healing process. People should allow themselves to be angry or upset when other people offer them what they see as patronising advice. There is no shame in sitting down and having a good cry because crying releases the body's endorphins, those natural salves of pain, both physical and emotional. Negative thoughts just bring on more negative thoughts and then you become trapped in a vicious circle of gloom. You should allow your-self to take comfort.

Many couples have told me that while they feel they are coping adequately with infertility, one small comment, or incident, can bring their deep-seated emotions flooding to the surface. Sadly, this will probably always happen. Realising the inevit-ability of this may make it easier for you to deal with it when it does. If one day you feel hurt allow yourself to cry or feel low. Talk about it with your partner. Don't feel you are failing because you can still feel hurt in this way.

Vivienne, who spoke to me about turning away from treatment, told me:

> It helps to have people around you who are supportive and non-judgmental. People *are* judgmental. There are lots of people who will tell you that if you can't have children, then that's the way it's meant to be. That sort of comment hurts even though you might be able to rationalise it.
>
> When people are sometimes insensitive, I don't think they really mean to hurt you. It's like talking about an illness; people feel they have to say something. Other people become really curious about why you can't have children. They want to know all the details about a really personal intimate sub-ject. They ask questions they wouldn't dream of asking someone who has no fertil-ity problems.

The pain of dealing with failed infertility treatment can be intense. For some couples the final realisa-tion that even IVF cannot offer them hope of a child can be far more devastating than they ever imagined. Some studies have shown that the stress of infertility is comparable to the stress suffered by people with cancer or a heart attack.

Elizabeth, a thirty-four-year-old personal assistant, has had four failed IVF attempts, but she still plans to keep on trying. She has blocked Fallopian tubes which surgery failed to improve.

> I was devastated when I was told I might not ever be able to have children. I couldn't even bear to think of life without them. My husband and I have so much love to give and I know I just won't feel whole without a child of my own.
>
> Each time I tried IVF and it failed I felt as though I was mourning for a lost child. For two weeks each time I totally believed I was pregnant and convinced myself I was pregnant. When I wasn't I hated myself. Why did it have to be me when all my friends had babies as easily as snapping their fingers? All the pain and suffering I have gone through and the years of treatment cannot be in vain.
>
> To me the pain of infertility is like an illness or an affliction that I will never be able to cope with. The only way for me to overcome it is to have a child. I cannot give up hope.

Joining a support group can be very beneficial in dealing with this pain. Much can be learned from the experience of others. Comfort and understanding gained from new friendships can be a help during weeks of waiting for hospital appointments or for the results of treatment. Talking to support-group members can be an enriching experience, because many couples find it difficult to discuss their problems with family or friends. Family and friends can be too close to the 'hurt'. Strangers can be more objective and simply easier to talk to as they're not involved.

There may be local support groups attached to your clinic. For details of two national support groups, ISSUE and CHILD, see page 102.

Some people find that reading as much as they can find on fertility and fertility treatments can help because they can keep up-to-date on all the latest developments. Support groups are invaluable for keeping members well informed.

Counselling is another way of seeking help. You can find out more about counselling from the associations mentioned on page 102. Assisted conception units which provide *in vitro* fertilisation and donor insemination are legally obliged to provide access to a trained independent counsellor for their patients (Human Fertilisation and Embryology Act, 1990).

People tell me that undergoing fertility treatment can feel like playing table tennis with your emotions, with people being batted to and fro between doctors, appointments, contradictory opinions, emotional highs and lows, insensitivity and often little continuity of care.

The waiting involved in NHS treatment has been difficult to deal with for Lisa and her husband Steve. Lisa, now thirty-six, first saw her GP about her failure to conceive when she was thirty-one.

The waiting for appointments has been really hard to deal with. There is such a gap between them that there seems to be no continuity in care. Every time I go in to the clinic there's a new face and the doctor has to read through my notes before asking me anything. It's very frustrating.

TURNING AWAY FROM TREATMENT

Some people find that they cannot give up the idea of a life without children until every possible aspect of their fertility problem has been fully investigated and no possible treatment left untried. Yet other people find that a decision to stop fertility treatment can be a major turning point for them. One person told me that she felt she had been given her life back, that she was now free – able to contemplate other issues in her life that she had neglected or that had been overshadowed by the constant interruptions that the treatment, with its attendant pain, frustration and disappointment, had caused.

Vivienne, a forty-two-year-old mother of two, experienced a great sense of relief when she and her husband decided to stop infertility treatment. They went on to adopt two children and have absolutely no regrets about the decision. She also believes she was fortunate in that she came to this decision in her mid twenties, rather than, as many couples do, leaving any thoughts about having children until their mid thirties.

> It was only because I'd had an ectopic pregnancy that I knew something was wrong. At least this gave me the chance to try for adoption, which would have been more difficult had I been older.
>
> Even so, I had infertility investigations for

three years. I had enough after that as it had begun to dominate my life. I had been the eternal optimist. I never thought I would not have children, but I was also never obsessed with having my own children in terms of actually wanting to give birth. I never thought that being obsessed was particularly productive. My husband had also been supportive and was always very easy to talk to about our fertility problems. He would always keep it fairly lighthearted, so it never got too intense.

Treatment started with all the usual tests to see if I was ovulating. I had to do temperature charts and take my temperature every day and I would feel awful if I forgot. You have to take it first thing when you wake up in the morning, so every day it's your first conscious thought and a reminder of your problem, which isn't very nice. Then waiting for your period to arrive and dealing with disappointment when it did. For me that wasn't that bad, but I had friends who went into a depression when a period arrived because it meant they were back on the treatment treadmill again.

My husband had to give sperm specimens. He didn't make a fuss about it – he just found it bizarre. Or I would be told this is the time you are most fertile and you have to make love at that point. You suddenly feel that this is what you ought to be doing rather than it being what you want to do. Having to make love makes the pleasure go out of it. It becomes terribly functional. For women it's possibly easier than for men.

I felt terrible for my husband because he had to perform on demand. I felt bad about him having to do that. When these feelings hit me I began to question whether it was really all worth it. It does put pressure on you and it does put pressure on a relationship. I began to wonder whether it was worth destroying a special relationship for something that might not work anyway.

While the staff you come in contact with may be helpful and nice, going to an infertility clinic is not a pleasant experience. There is little continuity in care, and you are made to feel like just a body, or a number, as so many people attend the clinic. But you feel that once you have started it you have got to go so far – until you discover what is wrong or until you decide you can't take any more of it. It is like a treadmill. It is also almost like being a child. You go to the clinic and they give you a little task to do each time you go. One week it's temperature charts, the next stage it will be hormones. You get the impression – which is probably true – that they are as much in the dark as you are and that it is a question of trial and error. It's as if you have to go through all sorts of processes so that the doctors can tick them off their list. It just seems so interminable when you are going through it. If I had been told at the start that this was the list of options I would have to go through, and how long it would take, it might have helped. I felt as if I was being treated as stupid.

The worst test of all for me was the post-coital test. Having to make love and then go in to the clinic destroys a certain amount of intimacy in your relationship. When you are examined after making love, it feels like a type of violation, apart from the embarrassment which you never get over. The process is not unpleasant. It's not painful. It's not even humiliating. It's just that you are laying yourself bare. It was after this that I began to think I didn't want to go on with it.

Vivienne also had two laparoscopies and a hysterosalpingogram, which she found extremely painful. She decided she could not deal with any more tests and explored adoption. 'When we decided to adopt it was a really big relief for me together with the thought that I didn't have to traipse back to the clinic and go through all the treatment rituals.'

Four years later she adopted a baby son. Following the adoption she had two more ectopic pregnancies and lost the second Fallopian tube. It was then she was offered IVF. She declined the treatment.

I already had my adopted son and thought that there was no big deal to giving birth. I didn't feel guilty for myself. I suppose I felt guilty for my husband. My husband had always been incredibly good. He never had a hang up about having his own genetic child – or if he did he never made me feel as if he did.

We also turned down a chance of IVF because of our adopted son. We felt it would be unfair to have one adopted child and one which was genetically ours. It seemed more sensitive to them to have two adopted children – not that you would have treated them differently. I feel absolutely that it was the right decision. Once you get past the first six months when everyone was talking about what their labour was like, I felt no different towards my children than if they were my own genetic children. After, say, six months what happened at the birth doesn't come into it – they are just your children.

ADOPTION

Adoption is one option for those who have fertility problems. But don't think that this is an easy option. Bringing up an adopted child is no different from bringing up your own genetic child. The emotional roller-coaster of being a parent will be just the same.

People's attitudes towards adoption have changed slightly in the last thirty years. For many adoptive parents the subject is no longer swathed in secrecy. Children are often told from an early age that they are adopted as it is believed that an open attitude rather than a secretive one is most helpful to the child.

If you want to find out more about adoption, a register of adoption agencies is available from the BAAF, British Agencies for Adoption and Fostering (see page 102 for details). Or you can contact the PPIAS, Parent to Parent Information on Adoption Services. PPIAS is able to help people who are considering adopting a child by passing on information about how and where to apply for adoption.

According to the BAAF there are black babies

waiting for black families and babies with dis-
abilities who need new homes. But if you are white
and have set your heart on adopting a healthy
white baby, you should be prepared for a long wait
and you should accept you may eventually be dis-
appointed as very few such children are available
for adoption.

The application process can be lengthy. You
need to understand from the outset that an adoption agency will want to establish a good working
relationship with you and you will need to
undergo medical examinations, to have personal
and police references, take part in discussion
preparation groups and to be interviewed
individually.

People tend not always to be prepared fully for
the lengthy process involved in adoption.
Vivienne, who talked about turning her back on infertility treatment on page 84, believes couples
need to think hard about what they might be up
against when they decide adoption would be the
right course to follow.

> We went through infertility treatment and
> then adoption. You can cope with anything
> after that because it puts your whole life
> under a microscope. Unless you go through
> it you have no perception of how you are
> scrutinised, how your relationship is scruti-
> nised. Looking back now, I feel that in some
> ways the selection process was probably a
> very good thing. It certainly makes you
> examine your motives very very hard. Our
> motives for having a child were all the usual
> ones like – I came from a large family and for

me a family wasn't a family without children. There were all the other ones too, like I
felt we had a lot to give a child. I suppose to
a certain extent I would not have felt complete unless I had become a mother. I felt we
had a lot to offer. And from a purely selfish
point of view because a child was what I
wanted.

Vivienne also believes that people need to realise
from the outset that they may have to wait a long
time before they finally have a child through adoption.

It took four years from discussing the option
to having a child. We had to wait more than
two years for a child after being accepted.
Any time after you have been accepted you
can be called on to accept a baby without
warning. The selection process and the waiting can put terrible pressure on a marriage.
We met several people in the course of all
the interviews. We know of some whose
marriages broke up because of the process
and the scrutiny. You are interviewed individually, you are interviewed as a couple
and while all this forces you to examine the
motives for adoption it can cause a rift between a couple.
    I was lucky in that I have cousins who are
adopted and to me adoption wasn't frightening. It didn't hold any fear. I know a lot of
people for whom it does. Often one half of
the couple feels it is second best to having
your own genetic child. We didn't think

that. We feel as much love for our children as if they were our genetic children.

We weren't obsessive about having a baby. A child has to be brought up normally, not brought up to become a little prince or a little princess. Especially after going through a long period of infertility treatment, I can understand how people fall into that way of thinking. I am sure it is the same for a lot of IVF babies – they are somehow even more precious than a baby conceived normally.

SURROGACY

Surrogacy, where a woman becomes pregnant and carries the baby-to-be for an infertile couple, is surrounded by controversy, yet this type of assisted reproduction technology is legal. However, it is illegal for the provider unit (the fertility clinic) to obtain or supply the services of the potential surrogate mother. For more information about surrogacy you can contact the COTS helpline on 01549 402401.

COMMON QUESTIONS

When is the best time to have a baby?
Apart from the health considerations, there are other factors to take into account in deciding when to have a baby. These factors, which can be even more complicated, may include your personal relationship, where and how you live, your career, financial situation, etc.

Many women approaching their thirties do feel pressurised to have a baby and start talking about the biological clock ticking away. Their mothers start saying they want to be grandmothers. Sometimes one partner is ready before another.

More and more women are having babies in their thirties and even forties.

While it is true that the risks of having a baby, say, at forty-five and the difficulties of conceiving at that age are greater from a physical point of view than they are for a woman in her twenties, modern obstetric care is now so good that if the baby was a wanted one and the parents were secure in their ability to care for the child, these small risks would be no deterrent.

I would say that the whole picture needs to be taken into consideration. It is not just a question of age; a would-be mother's overall health picture is usually the most important factor affecting the likelihood of conception and the success of a pregnancy, not purely the mother's age in isolation. So if you are in your late thirties or early forties and enjoy good health, age alone should not be a great risk factor. The problem is that a woman is at her most fertile in her mid twenties and fertility does start dropping after the age of thirty-five.

Will a miscarriage affect my chances of becoming pregnant again?

Many women who have had a miscarriage often worry that they will never be able to have a child or will become infertile. One writer once told me that she had two miscarriages in eighteen months, but investigations showed that there was no physical reason for this. The writer had also heard that miscarriages were caused by the body rejecting an abnormal foetus and she was subsequently worried that she would never produce a foetus that would grow into a normal baby.

A pregnancy that terminates naturally because of an abnormal foetus will usually do so very early on – within a few weeks of its start. Indeed, as many as one in five 'new' pregnancies may abort very early.

If miscarriages occur at a later stage, then mischance alone is likely to have caused them – an inexplicable interruption in the blood supply to the foetus being the main cause. This happens without any obvious reason and purely by chance in up to one in ten early miscarriages. And, the chances of it happening a second time with no explanation other than bad luck are one in a hundred. Therefore, very often there is every reason to look forward to another pregnancy with confidence and hope.

Do heavy periods indicate conception difficulties?

Providing a woman is still ovulating regularly there should not be any problems. The amount of blood flow during a menstrual period varies from woman to woman. Studies show that what one woman considers to be heavy may be considered light by another. The normal amount passed by individual healthy women varies in any case by between five ml (about one teaspoonful) and eighty ml (sixteen teaspoonfuls) at each period.

Will having a cone biopsy mean I won't be able to have a baby?

Cone biopsies worry many women. This procedure is carried out as a result of an abnormality following a cervical smear and many women are subsequently worried that it will prevent them conceiving.

When severely abnormal cells are discovered after a routine cervical smear, the specialist will usually look at the cervix using a colposcope – a microscope that can be focused from the outside on to the cervix. The cervix is then stained and the extent of the abnormal cells can be observed.

Specialists become skilled at knowing whether the extent of the abnormal cells is such that they can be removed with a laser, or whether a cone of the cervix around the entrance to the womb needs to be removed. This operation is known as a cone biopsy and it involves the removal of the abnormal surface cells as well as the tissue just below them which may be affected by abnormal cells.

A cone biopsy will not prevent conception. The carrying of the baby may be mildly less secure than before, but, in general, the chances are still heavily in favour that all will be well.

Can a vasectomy be reversed?

I occasionally receive letters from men who have had vasectomies during a first marriage. Sometimes there are instances when they marry for the second time and their new wife longs to have children. I am asked whether or not a man can become fertile again after a vasectomy.

The answer is it really depends when the man had the vasectomy. A vasectomy involves cutting or blocking the *vas deferens* – the tubes that carry sperm away from the testicles. The tubes lie just under the skin of the scrotum. If the procedure was within the last five years or so, then the two tubes, the *vas deferens*, are likely to have been severed in a way that should enable them to be rejoined successfully.

However, if the vasectomy was performed more than about two years ago, a change may have occurred in the sperm. So, even though the tubes can be rejoined and sperm can again be produced, the man's immune system – his antibodies – can have been brought in to play and now constantly bring about changes in the sperm so that they are no longer able to achieve conception. Therefore there is no guarantee that once a man's vasectomy has been reversed he will be able to produce a baby, although research shows that there is a good chance he will.

Can a failure to conceive be psychological?

This is a difficult one. Most doctors have seen couples for whom there appears to be no physical reason why they shouldn't conceive – and yet they don't. Understandably, many of these couples become tense, anxious and depressed. So the conclusion has often been drawn that this psychological effect is the reason for the continuing infertility. I believe it has a role to play, but I'd be hard put to prove this medically.

Can the size of a man's penis affect his fertility?
Possible infertility causes such anxiety that unfortunately almost every aspect of a man's
anatomy comes under scrutiny by some worried
partners. I have even been asked in the past about
whether or not the size of a man's penis has an
effect on his ability to father a child – a question
which may seem laughable but one which was
causing considerable distress to my correspon-
dent. With regard to penis size, we actually know
from the results of scientific examination that,
though the length of a man's non-erect penis can
vary quite considerably, such differences tend to
disappear when the penis is erect. The result is
that there is very little variation between the short-
est erect penis and the longest for men of the same
overall build. And, as for fathering a child, the fact
that an otherwise healthy man has a shorter-than-
average penis will not affect his fertility.

**Does following a reduced-calorie diet affect your
chances of conceiving?**
Women who have been dieting ask me about the
effect it might have on their fertility. I am regularly
asked if a strict calorie-controlled diet could in
some way be preventing them from conceiving.
The answer depends to what extent the woman is
cutting down on her food intake. A very low-
calorie diet will not necessarily stop you becoming
pregnant. Women in the world's famine areas do
conceive. However, it is true that a diet of this
severity could diminish your chances of becoming
pregnant – especially if your weight falls dramatically. In some women, ovulation, and also therefore
their periods, may stop if they go down to as little
as half a stone or so below their ideal weight. It is

as though nature is saying, 'I mustn't allow a pregnancy to occur – there's not enough food about to support it.' And if the woman does conceive, her baby would be extremely likely to have a lower birth weight than expected.

If a baby's weight dips below a certain point, general health problems are more likely to develop. Above all, women who are thinking about becoming pregnant must make sure that their diet is both adequate and balanced. Follow this advice and you will give yourself the best possible chance of getting pregnant – and of having a perfectly healthy baby.

Will having an abortion affect my chances of becoming pregnant in later life?

Sometimes women write to me asking whether they will be able to start a family even though they may have had a termination some years previously. Providing any such termination was straightforward then it should make no difference at all to the chances of conceiving.

Why are humans one of the most infertile of all mammals?

The reason for this is not completely understood. However, it is considered that it could be connected with the way women ovulate. Whereas most female animals – even our nearest animal 'relatives', the mammals – produce a number of eggs at the same time during their fertile cycle and this production is often triggered by sexual activity, the human female releases only one egg usually and only in the middle of her menstrual cycle. And whereas many mammals have a fertile time when they exude scents that make them particularly attractive sexually as well as accommodating to the male animal at that time, the human female doesn't have a similar physically-attracting mechanism at the time she ovulates, so that fertile time of the month may go unnoticed and thus the opportunity for conception may be missed. In addition, even when a human egg is fertilised there is still only between a one in four and a one in five chance of a baby developing.

Our two-year-old son was born as a result of artificial insemination by donor. Can you tell us whether he has the right to know that my husband is not his genetic father?
The answer is yes, in that your child now has the right to be told by the Human Fertilisation and Embryology Authority that he was conceived as a result of treatment using donated sperm or eggs. The authority is required by law to collect information from all licensed centres about every IVF and donor insemination in case children conceived in this way should wish to know something about their genetic background when they reach adulthood.

The HFEA needs to know the name and date of birth of sperm donors in order to safeguard the interests of children born as a result of donor insemination. The HFEA says that people aged sixteen or over, who ask, can be told whether they could be related to someone they want to marry. Without basic identifying information, such as name and age, the authority could not establish whether or not there is a genetic relationship between people who wish to marry. Fulfilling this legal duty will not involve the disclosure of any information about the donor.

I am currently undergoing IVF treatment. Can you tell me what happens to 'spare' embryos from treatment?

When hormone drugs are used to stimulate egg production in the ovaries, more than three eggs (the maximum allowed for subsequent transfer) are usually collected and fertilised. The remaining embryos can be frozen for use in future treatments. Embryos can be stored for a maximum of five years. You do also have the option of donating the stored embryos, or collected eggs, for another woman to use in treatment or for research purposes.

At what age does a man become too old to father a child?

Charlie Chaplin became a father in his eighties and the oldest father ever recorded was 104! As you can see, there is no age limit for a man in good health.

While probably one in three women cannot conceive over the age of forty, many men are still quite fertile in their sixties. Some Canadian research suggested that men over forty-five produce far more defective sperm than younger men.

CONCERNS ABOUT INFERTILITY TREATMENT

Infertility treatment opens up so many questions for would-be parents. Should you tell your child he or she was conceived as a result of donor insemination? Even the advent of a revolutionary technique, such as ICSI, can cause a dilemma for couples who might already have one child as a result of donor insemination and who want to enlarge their family. Should the first child be told he or she has different genetic origins from the second? Should we be allowed to choose the sex of our children? Sex selection seems to be acceptable for medical reasons where a woman could have a baby with a life-threatening, sex-linked disease such as a certain sort of muscular dystrophy or haemophilia, but not just because of preferred choice. Should there be an upper age limit for fertility treatment? Should you be offered IVF treatment in return for egg donation? Questions develop and assume huge dimensions, incorporating ethical dilemmas such as whether donated ovarian tissue, including tissue from aborted foetuses should be used in infertility treatment and research. The list of questions could be endless.

And because of the very strong drive for couples to have their own baby, there is more of an opportunity for fertility services to become 'big business', with the attendant potential for exploitation. There are worries about a couple bringing pressure to bear upon the provider of such a service, for example, to 'order' a pregnancy of a particular sex. This unnatural selection, if it was allowed, could possibly have unforeseen consequences for all of us. There are also the potential problems involved in a woman donating eggs to another woman; about implanting so many embryos that there are too many multiple births with triplets, for example, being produced. What are the consequences of terminating some of the developing foetuses if the couple decide they don't want triplets, and so wish one or two of them to be aborted? And should a woman who has passed the menopause – the natural end to her child-bearing years – be offered the modern techniques that can once more allow her to carry a pregnancy? Should we be meddling with nature in any case? Should we be spending so much time and effort pursuing fertility techniques when much of the world is overcrowded and still plagued with disease – shouldn't we be treating the diseases first?

You can see that there are many ethical questions that remain unanswered. I believe that the rapidity of our discoveries in only the last two decades is the main reason for our ethical 'insecurities' and that, given acceptable guidelines, we shall soon feel easier about these issues.

So where, at present, do we draw the line? Strictly controlled research is vital if we are to make progress, particularly in the realm of genetic defects, but also to find out more about congenital disease and the cause of miscarriage. No doubt new developments will produce more ethical questions for us to consider.

USEFUL ADDRESSES

BAC, British Association for Counselling, 1 Regents Place, Rugby CV21 2DJ. Telephone: 01788 578328.

BAAF, British Agencies for Adoption and Fostering, Skyline House, 200 Union Street, London SE1 0LY. Telephone: 0171 593 2000.

BICA, The British Infertility Counselling Association, The White House, High Street, Campsall, Doncaster DN6 9AF. Telephone: 01302 701128.

CHILD, Charter House, 43 St Leonards Road, Bexhill-on-Sea, East Sussex TN40 1JA. Twenty-four-hour helpline: 01424 732361.

HFEA, The Human Fertilisation & Embryology Authority, Paxton House, 30 Artillery Lane, London E1 7LS. Telephone: 0171 377 5077.

ISSUE, The National Fertility Association, 509 Aldridge Road, Great Barr, Birmingham B44 8NA. Telephone: 0121 344 4414 (twenty-four hours with answerphone).

NEEDS, National Egg and Embryo Donation Society, Regional IVF Unit, St Mary's Hospital, Whitworth Park, Manchester M13 0JH. Telephone: 0161 276 6000.

The National Infertility Awareness Campaign. For a free information pack call Freephone 0800 716345.

AUSTRALIA
ACCESS, Australia's National Infertility Network represents the national interests of 47 infertility self-help groups around Australia.

Adoptive Parents Association of Canberra Inc, PO Box 1030, Woden, ACT 2606, Australia.
International Federation of Infertility Patient Associations, BOX 959, Parramatta NSW 2124, Australia. Telephone: 61 2 670 2380.

CANADA
Adoption Options, 10508 – 82 Avenue, Edmonton, Alberta, Canada, T6E 2A4.

IAAC, The Infertility Awareness Association of Canada Inc. This is the only organisation at national level providing increased awareness of infertility as well as support at local level in the direct delivery of service programmes.

INDEX